500 Tips For Coping With Chronic Illness

written and compiled by

Pamela D. Jacobs, M.A.

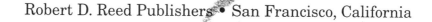

Robert D. Reed Publishers • San Francisco, California

Robert D. Reed Publishers & Pamela D. Jacobs Publishing

750 La Playa, Suite 647 • San Francisco, CA 94121
Telephone: (415) 997-4567 • Fax: (415) 997-3800

Book Cover by Destiny Design, PDJ, and Joseph E. Haga
Cover Photo, Book Design, and Typesetting by Pamela D. Jacobs
Editing by Susan Cattoche, Ann Jacobs, Nancy Schlesinger, and Darlene Frank
Layout by Heather Havrilesky

Library of Congress Cataloging-in-Publication Data

Jacobs, Pamela D.
    500 tips for coping with chronic illness / by Pamela D. Jacobs.
        p.   cm.
    Includes bibliographical references.
    1. Chronic diseases—Popular works. I. Adjustment (Psychology)—Popular works.
I. Title. II. Title: Five hundred tips for coping with chronic illness.
RC108.J33   1994
616'.001'9—dc20   94-16785
ISBN 1-885003-04-8 : $11.95   CIP

Designed, Typeset, Printed, and Manufactured in the United States of America.

* * *

To **Bob Reed**,
an "endangered species."
Thanks for making the world
a brighter, more colorful place.

Contents

Acknowledgments

I wish to express appreciation for the generous support of the following people:

To my partner and publisher, **Robert D. Reed**, for his integrity, strength, and uplifting sense of humor. I appreciate his great contribution to this book and to my life, and I respect his ongoing humanitarian and environmental efforts.

To my parents, **Annibelle** and **Sid**, and to my three wonderful brothers, **Larry**, **Steve**, and **Stan**, for their love and encouragement, and for being there 100%.

To **Megan**, **Nicholas**, **Emily**, **Sharon, Naomi**, **Sara**, **Darren, Jamie,** and **Kyley Jacobs**; **Julie Parker**; and **Shig Marumoto**—my family. And to **Catherine Taylor, Pat Engel**, **Liz Chickering**, **Mikel Bryant**, **Lenka Studnickova**; **Catherine**, **Helga**, and **Doug Carlton**; and to **Blythe** and **Land Wilson**—my "family in spirit."

To **Valerie Hearn, Ph.D.** for her contribution to the psychological and emotional health sections in this book. To **Martin Borge**, **D.C.** for his input and consultations. To **Ellen Raskin** for Qi Gong lessons and health care support. To massage therapist, **Kathy Jacobson**, for references and healing massages, and to her partner-in-healing, **Joyce Van Horn**, for providing a guiding light.

My sincere thanks to the following people for their support and contributions:

To **Harold J. Kristal, D.D.S.**, **William Lockyer, M.D.**, and **Jeffry Anderson, M.D.** for their help, consultations, and encouragement. And to **Preston Peña** and **David Mon** for their ongoing support of my work.

To **Heather Havrilesky**, **Ann Jacobs**, **Susan Cattoche**, and **Nancy Schlesinger**, for their assistance with my book. To **John Gray, Ph.D.** for permission to reprint material from his book, *What You Feel You Can Heal* (Heart Publishing, 1994). And to **Richard Leviton**, editor of Future Medicine Publishing, for permission to reprint material from *Alternative Medicine* (1993).

To **Marian Bernstein**, lecturer of Classical Archaeology and Museum Studies at San Francisco State University, and **Darlene Frank**, instructional designer, for their inspirational and enthusiastic guidance in the technical writing field.

To **Penny Snyder** and **Stan Smith**, at The School of Actualism, for their expertise in teaching a healing form of meditation, using color and light energy. And to **Rev. Stan Hampson** at Unity Church in Palo Alto, and **Rev. Sharon Connors** at Unity in San Francisco, for teaching the healing power of prayer.

My thanks to **Mark Gillham** and **Joseph Haga** for designing and producing the book cover and for incorporating my photograph of waterlilies from the botanical gardens in Niagara Falls, Canada. (In many cultures, waterlilies and lotus blossoms represent sacred symbols of healing life energy and eternal life.)

Finally, I would like to express my appreciation for all of the courageous women and men in our support group meetings—people who continue to share their experiences, strength, compassion, honesty, and unconditional love to help others.

Note To The Reader

This book is for people who are dealing with chronic illness, whether they are experiencing illness or caring for loved ones who are ill. Students and professionals in the fields of health and psychology may also find it beneficial.

Writing a book is a huge undertaking and a challenge for anyone. It has been especially difficult for me to write this book while I was dealing with an illness that causes fatigue. I was also editing four other books and trying to maintain my life. Yet this book is "living proof" that if I could accomplish this goal under these conditions, then you, too, can achieve your goals using similar methods: by taking one step at a time, balancing work with rest and health care, getting support, setting up a clear plan and a flexible schedule, and being determined.

There's a wonderful expression: "We teach what we most need to learn." Writing *500 Tips For Coping With Chronic Illness* has been a big lesson for me, one that I want to share with those who face similar challenges. It has made me confront and move beyond my limitations and has taught me to set healthier boundaries. It has forced me to grow, deal with fears (such as fear of criticism) and overcome major obstacles (such as severe writer's block). There were times when researching and writing this book was so overwhelming that I considered renaming it: *500 Tips For **NOT** Coping With Chronic Illness*.

Some days, as I struggled to sort through research materials or forced myself to sit down and write, I wondered if I were the right person to write about coping with illness. Yet these experiences led me to an important discovery. I realized that "coping" is a learning process, a natural part of everyone's life. On some days, people may not feel like coping...and that's OK. Making that OK takes some of the pressure off. Remember that even healthy people do not function at their peak levels one hundred percent of the time. We all need a little "down time" for rejuvenating and letting off steam. And we need to let go of trying to control everything, which is an immense burden. Having an "escape valve" on the pressure cooker of our lives can help us to create breakthroughs instead of breakdowns. One effective coping statement that I have found useful is: "Each day, I am doing the *best* that I can." Try saying this whenever you feel that you are not living up to your own expectations! And do yourself a favor... Forget about living up to the expectations of others.

Coping with illness is similar to taking a few steps forward, moving a few steps back, and then pushing forward again. Seeing the whole picture of our lives provides a healthy perspective. We can lighten up about problems and see the positive aspects, along with the negative. The key is to let go and have fun with the steps forward, backward, and forward. We can call it the "Coping Two-Step" and enjoy the dance. With this enlightened attitude, we increase our chances of having more good days than bad—which is our goal.

Writing this book has taught me how to surmount obstacles, both real and imagined. This work has been similar to researching and writing my master's thesis, a catalog of ancient Egyptian artifacts. Both subjects (Egyptology and health) involve an in-depth exploration of human nature (the body, mind, heart, and soul). They cover topics such as history, medicine, science, technology, art, language, literature, psychology, philosophy, spirituality, and the After-life.

Coping with illness is a highly complex issue. It took several years to research and gather information for this book. It was challenging (and fascinating!) to sort through thousands of books, articles, and reference materials, as well as to review my notes from lectures, medical conferences, support groups, and consultations with doctors and people living with illness. I have also compiled personal tips (discovered by trial and error), which have helped to enhance my own healing. The good news is that there are thousands of resources for coping. And there are thousands of ways in which people can be effective and nurturing caregivers. *500 Tips...* provides only a glimpse of available resources and ideas.

Finally, I was able to complete this book by staying focused on my primary goal: the desire to share with you what has worked for me and others in our healing process so that you may be inspired to find support or information when you need to brighten your outlook, uplift your spirit, or get medical care.

Foreword

by Valerie Hearn, Ph.D.

Chronic illness, like any challenge of life, necessitates the development of new coping skills. What does "coping" mean? In this delightful and sensible book, Pamela Jacobs has drawn on her own and others' experiences to show us that while coping may mean accepting what cannot be changed, coping also means taking action. It means doing what you can do and taking charge of the things that you can change.

Since stress usually accompanies chronic illness, the sections in this book on promoting psychological and emotional health are especially welcome. Cognitive therapy is now the treatment of choice for many difficulties (including depression and stress-related problems) that besiege Americans today. One of the basic tenets of cognitive therapy is that stress is determined not by what happens to you but by the way you think about and respond to your experience. The stress that accompanies a long-term illness can be made far worse by habitual negative ways of thinking which do not take into account many options simply because one has never thought of them. This "tunnel vision" leads to feeling bad and creates self-defeating ways of behaving.

500 Tips For Coping With Chronic Illness offers many excellent suggestions for changing the way you think about your state of health—offering positive, action-oriented behavioral and psychological options which can reduce stress, create a more hopeful outlook, and ultimately improve health.

This book also provides hundreds of practical, creative ideas for dealing with other aspects of life—from financial to social to spiritual. In addition, the "Resources for Help & Information" section offers a wealth of useful suggestions. *500 Tips...* is an invaluable guide for coping with living, whether you are sick or well.

Preface

What are the most effective ways to cope with chronic illness? After years of living with illness, I would highly recommend these basic survival techniques:

- Develop a solid foundation for coping by building a network of support.
- Raise your self-esteem by loving yourself unconditionally.
- Actively participate in your own healing process.
- Incorporate simple healing activities into all areas of your life: physical, psychological, emotional, spiritual, and social.

Here are some examples:

Physical Health
Pay attention to how your body feels.
Schedule activities according to your energy level.
Create harmony and balance in your life.
Get appropriate exercise. Go for a walk and breathe fresh air.

Psychological Health
Develop a positive attitude, healthy self image, self-love, and respect.
Pay attention to your thoughts, both positive and negative.

Set healthy limits for yourself and others.
Work with a caring therapist who specializes in coping with illness.

Emotional Health
Maintain a sense of humor. Laughter is good for your immune system.
Try to have some fun every day.
Watch a funny movie.
Sing your favorite songs.
Join a support group. And find a telephone support person.

Spiritual Health
Have faith. Pray and ask for strength and healing.
Be at peace with life.
Feel a spiritual connection to the Universe.
Ask your angels for healing guidance.

Social Health
Spend more time with children.
Give and receive plenty of hugs and "tender loving care."
Be open and honest with yourself and others.
Get help to heal any family conflicts.
Tell your loved ones often that you love them.

A powerful saying that may offer you encouragement is: "God does not give challenges to people who cannot handle them." Begin to think of yourself as a strong person, one who can work through obstacles and achieve your goals. Take good care of yourself every day and you will experience numerous rewards.

With many chronic illnesses, traditional medical care and treatments may not always provide a complete cure. Health care providers sometimes do not offer the understanding we need. Taking charge of your own healing and health care can help to empower you. Reach out, talk to others, read, become informed about your illness, and find appropriate help and support. Fortunately, we live in a rich and diverse culture where support is alive and well. With the right help and resources, anyone (yes, even *you*) can handle any challenge life offers.

Wishing you improved health and vitality.

– *Pamela D. Jacobs*
San Francisco, California

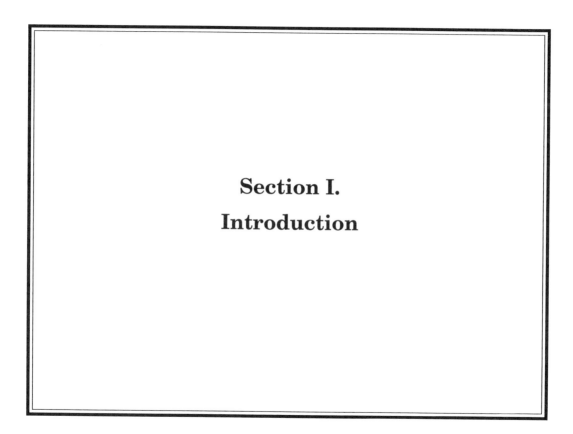

Section I.
Introduction

Introduction

500 Tips For Coping With Chronic Illness is a resource guide, providing a general overview of suggestions, information, ideas, books, and other materials that have helped me and hundreds of others with our healing, discovery, and recovery. The goal of this book is to encourage and empower those who live with illness and to offer support to caregivers. The tips deal with various aspects of life—from healing the body, mind, heart, and soul—to finding alternative ways to earn extra money. Select only ideas which will be beneficial to you and discuss them with your doctor, therapist, support group, family, or friends. Be sure to check with your doctor before beginning any program that affects your health.

This book is based on my personal experiences with chronic illness for sixteen years and many years of research—including my talks with hundreds of people who live with debilitating health conditions; consultations with medical doctors and holistic health professionals; facilitating support groups for people with chronic illness; answering hotline calls; attending health classes, lectures, and medical conferences; and developing resources and appropriate referrals.

In the "Recommended Reading & Tapes" section, I have provided a list of some of the most nurturing and supportive materials available today. Reading and learning about health, listening to healing tapes, cooking healthful meals, and nurturing yourself are just *some* of the "500 Tips" recommended for well-being.

A Personal Journey—From Illness To Wellness

In the late 1970s, I was finally able to leave a six-year relationship that had become extremely abusive. After recuperating for several months and beginning a new life, I came down with a severe flu which lingered on and on. Daily low-grade fevers, exhaustion, and muscle weakness made it increasingly difficult to work, attend school, and keep up with my social life. This was frustrating because I had always been fit, healthy, and active. My energy continued to decline. Some days, I'd get up, take a shower, get dressed...but fatigue forced me to cancel my plans and go back to bed. It became obvious that I needed some medical help.

One doctor at a health maintenance organization ordered several standard tests, but these tests revealed nothing "abnormal." The doctor said, "Everything's fine. In fact, you have a *glowing* medical report." While I was grateful to hear that nothing appeared to be wrong, I still felt ill and in need of treatment. Little did I know that this was only the beginning of my long search for medical answers. Over time, I discovered that my illness was not widely recognized or understood by most people, including doctors. Not only was I faced with challenges associated with chronic illness, I also had to find information and a doctor who could help.

Finally, in 1989 (after eleven years and numerous tests), my big break came when a doctor diagnosed my condition as Chronic Fatigue Immune Dysfunction Syndrome (CFIDS), also known as Chronic Fatigue Syndrome (CFS). Naturally, I assumed that a diagnosis would lead to a cure. Unfortunately, I was wrong.

The cause and effective treatment of CFS are presently unknown. Symptoms, which tend to wax and wane, may include low energy, disabling fatigue (especially after exercise), fevers, flu-like symptoms, pain, muscle weakness, and more.

Neil F. Gordon, M.D., of the Cooper Clinic and Research Institute and author of *Chronic Fatigue: Your Complete Exercise Guide* (Human Kinetics Publishers, 1993), writes:"Whether a CFS patient is young or old, the disease causes similar hardships. CFS is a debilitator that can trigger a whole host of human relations problems. Indeed, one of the worst things about the condition is its negative effect on people's lives. Even a moderate case of CFS can destroy a person's ability to be productive and fully functional. Another problem is finding a doctor with adequate knowledge of the CFS puzzle and experience with CFS patients.... Those with the ill fortune to consult a nay-saying or unsympathetic physician may end up doctor-shopping. And whether the end result of this unfortunate practice is satisfactory or not, there's one guaranteed outcome—staggering bills."

Chronic Fatigue Syndrome has not been taken seriously by many physicians; some still refuse to acknowledge it. Several doctors implied that my symptoms were "all in my head." One doctor rushed into the examining room, shaking my chart at me and yelling, "What do you want from me? Why are you here? I don't even *believe* in Chronic Fatigue Syndrome!" (as if it were a religion). Calmly, I replied, "You *would* believe in it if you had it." This experience, among others, motivated me to write this book. It is hard enough to deal with a serious illness and its impact on your life. No one should have to suffer additional trauma and humiliation by being invalidated or verbally abused. My hope is to encourage readers to find and accept only compassionate and professional medical care.

The most difficult challenge I've had dealing with chronic illness has been the tremendous skepticism of some doctors, friends, colleagues, and even family members. For some reason, they have not believed that I was physically ill. They'd say, "But, you *look* fine!" (implying I was only imagining things or was a hypochondriac). Well, *looks* can be deceiving with some illnesses. While I have continued to do everything possible to rebuild my energy and well-being, I no longer have the patience or desire to convince others about my state of health.

Fortunately, today, CFS is more accepted as a "legitimate" illness and disability. Doctors, scientists, and the Centers For Disease Control are involved with research. Since the first CFS conference in San Francisco in 1989, there have been annual international medical conferences on this illness. And I have been able to meet hundreds of people with similar symptoms and experiences. We have developed a strong network of support to share information and referrals.

After too many years of experiencing illness, I have learned some valuable tips that I enjoy sharing with others. First, I believe that it is vital (for our physical, mental, and emotional health) to remain as active, productive, and social as possible. I have also learned how important it is to get plenty of rest to build a reserve of energy for healing. Remaining optimistic has also contributed to my healing process, as has finding the right lifestyle, nutrition, exercise, doctor, and treatment. Continuing to pursue personal and professional goals has enhanced my self-esteem as well as my outlook. Determination has allowed me to do film production work, to complete a graduate degree, and to write and edit books, scripts, and marketing materials. Several people with similar health problems have asked me, "How can you go to school or write a book? I can't even walk to the store or write a letter!" I've replied, "By taking one step (or writing one page) at a time, we can achieve almost anything. Persistence and a sense of humor are effective tools for staying motivated through the toughest times."

Establishing and working toward healthy personal goals, while dealing with chronic illness, can help to uplift our spirits as well as our self-esteem. Focusing on a goal, whether large or small, can make us feel better mentally and physically. Our goals can be as simple as reading a book, learning something new, painting a picture, going for a walk, or planting a few seeds in a garden. Being involved in pleasurable activities is rejuvenating for the body, mind, heart, and soul.

Working toward a goal while coping with illness requires paying attention to how you feel. Your goal should be appropriate for your condition. You may need to consult with your doctor before beginning a new project. Remember to balance any work or hobby with plenty of rest. By setting up a flexible schedule and by carefully pacing yourself, you can achieve almost any goal you desire. Taking frequent breaks, meditating, getting a massage, or doing some physical therapy exercises are good ways to nurture yourself. Finding the right resources, being optimistic, having patience with yourself, and setting up a support network are all good coping tips. Learn to ask for help when you need it, and don't feel guilty about asking for help. One effective way to move beyond guilt is to help others as you help yourself. Offering encouragement to someone, or just listening to someone who needs to talk, can give you a sense of purpose and accomplishment.

One of my goals for writing this book is to prevent others who are ill from going through similar frustrations that I have experienced while living with chronic illness in our fast-paced, action- and money-oriented society. Let's face it, illness is a subject that most people do not want to hear about or discuss. However, we can all benefit from having more compassion for and understanding of those who are ill. Like it or not, illness is a part of life. Accepting that fact can help us to prepare for the realities of illness when we are suddenly faced with it, or when we have a loved one who becomes ill.

Although it often pulls the rug out from under us, illness can also force us to make constructive changes. While illness may close some doors, it can also open up new ones. Illness can encourage us to re-evaluate ourselves and our lives, pointing us in new and positive directions. It can motivate us to listen more carefully to our inner selves, while inspiring us to reach out to those who are near and dear to us. Sharing our feelings and personal experiences, both positive and negative, often serves a higher purpose. Expressing our knowledge and strengths may help to inform or support others in profound ways. Shifting our focus from personal health problems to helping others can empower us while also preventing isolation. Sharing our unique ideas for handling difficult situations may help save lives.

Many people tend to be in denial about illness—never fully preparing for the possibility of becoming ill (beyond establishing health insurance or stocking up on over-the-counter drugs for sleep, a lift, or a cold). People assume that serious illness just won't effect them. But, whether sick or well, everyone can benefit by practicing preventive health care. Making healthy choices about our nutrition, exercise, and lifestyle are among our most important decisions.

Some people are uncomfortable dealing with others who are chronically ill. Well-meaning family members may not know what to say or how to help relatives with health problems. Employers may become angry if an employee is forced to take extensive time off because of illness. Even some doctors become frustrated with patients who do not respond to treatment and may eventually refuse to treat them. (Unfortunately, I have seen this happen!) To make matters worse, chronic illness can cause feelings of discouragement or isolation. So it is essential to find support for coping with these overwhelming feelings and experiences.

Reaching out for help and helping others is empowering. Many people who contacted me for advice and support have offered information and support in return. Helping others can have a positive "snowball" effect. That is why support groups are so effective and popular. When people get together over time, sharing their feelings, comparing experiences, and working toward common goals, they develop strength as a group and as individuals. There *is* "strength in numbers." Knowing that you are not alone can comfort you and give you hope.

After being ill for months or years, people commonly experience feelings of hopelessness and helplessness. It is important to discuss these feelings with someone. If you are able to share your strength and resources (simply by listening, caring, or providing a little light at the end of the tunnel), it is a rewarding (and sometimes lifesaving) act of kindness. When someone expresses his or her appreciation of your help and understanding, it can make you feel good. The more we help each other feel comfortable, the more we experience peace. Note: If people reach out to you when they are feeling suicidal, call a doctor or Suicide Prevention. Take them seriously.

To cope with a chronic illness, focus on what you *can* do; let go of what you can no longer do. Just shifting perspectives from one of "doom and gloom" to one of "hope and optimism" can have an uplifting effect. Hope can be a connection to our spirit, our will to live, and our life energy for healing. The body responds to thoughts, whether positive or negative. Feeling hopeless can lead to destructive thoughts and actions, whereas positive thoughts and feelings promote healing.

Chronic illness can often devastate one's work and financial security. Therefore, establishing new ways to earn money can be essential for coping and maintaining income and peace of mind. This book includes alternative ways to earn money when illness prevents you from working full-time. There are many things you may consider. For example, developing a home-based business on a flexible schedule is one way you can earn money while dealing with illness or disability. Remember, no one can fire you for calling in sick because *you* are the boss.

At times chronic illness can alter your entire life. I have met people who have lost their strength, athletic abilities, careers, income, security, homes, cars, marriages, relationships, hobbies, creativity, ability to concentrate, and even their health insurance! One doctor, who suffers from chronic fatigue syndrome said, "There is *nothing* that this illness cannot take away from you."

After years of being productive and social, anyone would find it difficult to deal with pain, loss, isolation, and limitations. Illness can have a great impact on our mental well-being. We need time to accept and adjust to the loss of our former, more productive lifestyles. So it is crucial to get appropriate help. In fact, the right support at the right time can save lives—maybe even your own.

Many people with serious conditions have found that their illnesses forced them to create healthier lifestyles. They slowed down and focused on what was most important to them. Some people spent more time with their children, some became involved with new hobbies, and others began exercising and walking more. Eventually, they felt better as they developed a new appreciation for life. In most cases, their new attitude was a turning point toward improved health.

Doctors with whom I consulted recommended these healthy suggestions:

For the body: Make healthier lifestyle choices. Eat nutritious foods and drink plenty of fresh water. Build strength and boost the immune system. Take supplements and herbs as recommended by your doctor or nutritionist— such as vitamin C, B-complex, trace minerals, and Ginseng. Plant enzymes may help to improve digestion and nutritional absorption. Limit sugar, fats, alcohol, caffeine, and smoking. Avoid exposure to chemicals. Do some form of regular exercise. Get a massage or do self-massage. Take naps when needed.

For the mind: Find a supportive therapist. Meditate. Think positive thoughts. Laugh hard and often. Reduce stress. Be creative. Resolve conflicts.

For the heart: Spend more quality time with your loved ones. Resolve interpersonal conflicts. Share your feelings. Develop a support network.

<u>For the soul</u>: Attend a service that uplifts you and makes you feel good. Pray. Read the Scriptures or a spiritual book. Make a list of inspirational quotes.

Becoming more dedicated to improving my health has also created a healthier life for me. I have finally established a committed, nurturing relationship with a man who loves and accepts me unconditionally. Our high-quality relationship has enhanced my well-being and self-esteem. Now whenever I talk to women about the importance of having a healthy relationship, especially those living with chronic illness, I can speak from personal experience and say it is possible!

Having a supportive family, close friends, a caring therapist, and a positive support network have all had a healing effect. Thankfully, my sense of humor has remained intact. It is an effective survival tool. I have also been inspired by healing workshops, insightful books, uplifting films, comedy shows, walks by the ocean, interesting classes, creative projects, spiritual teachers, and prayer. All of these holistic activities have contributed to a happier, more balanced life.

Over the years, I have met hundreds of people with chronic illness—at medical conferences, lectures, support groups, hospitals, and libraries. Most of them are bright, talented, brave, compassionate, and loving; some of them have become close friends. If I had never experienced chronic illness, I may have missed meeting these inspiring people. For this reason, I do not regret my challenges.

Another important challenge for coping with illness is to establish new sources of income. When illness forced me to leave my work in film production, I was devastated! I could no longer work long hours every day. Eventually I set up a part-time writing business at home, which ultimately turned out to be a blessing. Writing is aligned with my career goals. My M.A. degree is in writing, and it is exciting to build a business in this field. So while illness forced me to give up work I loved, it also led me to create new work and a more appropriate schedule. Philosophically, it helped to take Joseph Campbell's advice, "Follow your bliss and doors will open for you...." And doors did open. I found writing/editing work, including work on screenplays, and I met authors, publishers, and producers at workshops. Maybe it was my fate to live with chronic illness, as the experience of learning to cope has provided a basis for writing and assisting others who are ill. By coming to terms with illness, I am making it an ally instead of an enemy. By working around my limitations, I am reducing stress, making peace with my past and present life, and I am thinking more optimistically about the future.

Fortunately, humans are blessed with an incredible ability to adapt when faced with illness, pain, suffering, loss, grief, or hardship. Amazingly, we've developed ways to cope, manage, adjust, bounce back, and thrive under difficult conditions. We can even get help to strengthen our determination and develop our courage. While this evolutionary process may not be fun or easy, it's a relief to know that it is possible to surmount obstacles and create healthier work and lifestyles.

Section II.
500 Tips For Coping With Chronic Illness

<u>Notes To The Reader:</u>

A)   The following pages offer a wide range of tips for coping with personal health challenges. One important tip is this: If you ever feel overwhelmed trying to cope all by yourself, reach out and ask for help. There are countless resources and organizations in this country. And there are many qualified, compassionate, and caring professionals to support your healing efforts.

B)   Obviously, not all of the following tips and ideas will be appropriate for everyone. Therefore, choose **only** the suggestions that feel right for you and then talk with your doctor, therapist, or caregiver about them.

C)   To organize this book, I have divided it into sections on promoting physical, psychological, emotional, and spiritual health. Naturally, all of these areas are interrelated, and many tips reflect this interrelationship.

Chapter 1. Life Management Tips For
Healing Your Body, Mind, Heart & Soul

Ancient healers and philosophers believed that the mind and body were one. Modern research confirms this mind/body connection. Studies show that an optimistic outlook can improve physical health and stimulate a healing response. Laughter can boost the immune system by releasing endorphins. Your emotions can also have a direct impact on physiological states. Negative feelings can cause stress, anxiety, and illness; while joy and love can uplift you and promote well-being. Prayer has been demonstrated to play an important role in healing the mind and body. Therefore, the key to improving your health is to balance love, laughter, proper nutrition, exercise, work, and spirituality in your life.

In his book, *Healing And The Mind*, Bill Moyers interviews physicians, scientists, therapists, and patients—people who are taking a new look at the meaning of sickness and health. He discusses their search for answers to perplexing questions, such as: How do emotions translate into chemicals in our bodies? How do thoughts and feelings influence health? How can we help our bodies to heal? The book reveals how advances in mind/body medicine are being applied in the world of modern medicine. "From neonatal care to geriatrics, from surgery to treatment of chronic illness, medical professionals are finding that when they practice the 'new medicine,' their patients heal faster, leave the hospital sooner, and do better once they get home." Moyers' documentary film, "Healing And The Mind" (which was shown on PBS), explores numerous benefits of Western medicine, Chinese medicine, and alternative therapies.

Bernie Siegel, M.D. (a surgeon in New Haven, Connecticutt, a teacher at Yale University, and author of *Love, Medicine & Miracles* and *Peace, Love & Healing)*, writes about "exceptional cancer patients" and the human ability to adapt to living with illness. He has seen firsthand how one's attitude, emotions, beliefs, and will-to-live can heal. He is convinced that healing begins with self-love.

Norman Cousins, author of *Anatomy of an Illness*, wrote: "Eighty-five percent of all illness is self-limiting. Your body, if given rest and good nutrition, is designed to heal itself of most illnesses. Nature, time, and patience are the three great physicians." He suggested that deep laughter (or "inner jogging") is highly beneficial for boosting immunity and health.

The insightful, informative, and inspirational books (mentioned above and throughout this book) explore various aspects of human health—from the inside out and the outside in. Self-help (or "shelf" help) books cover a wide range of healing options and techniques from A to Z—from aging gracefully to zestful living. You have probably already experienced how reading and sharing healing books and articles can enlighten, entertain, and empower you and loved ones.

Healthy Perspectives

Reverend Stan Hampson, at Unity Church in Palo Alto, California says, "By being honest, building up our energy, accepting and loving ourselves and others, and by developing trust, faith, and hope, we support the healing process in our body, mind, heart, and spirit." He provides this positive formula for healing:

H	—	Honesty
E	—	Energy
A	—	Acceptance
L	—	Love
T	—	Trust
H	—	Hope

Reverend Hampson states, "We change in an environment of love, not criticism. The world changes as we make changes. Peace on earth begins within, for our thoughts create our physical reality. We can decide our reactions, instead of being compulsive or obsessive. We can organize our problems, instead of globalizing or agonizing over them. We can decide what to do, and then do it. Finally, we can hold on to faith for strength and healing."

In China, doctors are paid to keep people well. When people become ill they stop paying for medical care until they get well again. Acupuncture and other traditional forms of medicine are used only after patients have been encouraged to create more harmony in their lives. Creating balance is the first step to healing.

In the United States, making significant lifestyle changes and getting our lives into balance is challenging—mainly because we tend to be focused outward. For example, we tend to turn on our television sets more often than we let our imaginations entertain or heal us. Generally, we are not trained from childhood to meditate or to be in harmony with nature. Most of us get caught up living life in the fast lane and it is hard to slow down. Workaholic behavior has become more prevalent, especially during tough economic times. Workaholism is considered a virtue by many people, especially employers. But without an appropriate balance of work and relaxation, a high-powered lifestyle can lead to stress and *dis*-ease. Being still and focusing inward seems almost foreign to most of us. However, this process is fundamental to our health and well-being.

Setting new priorities and goals is a good way for you to begin a program for coping with chronic illness. Your illness may be "signaling" you to change how you think, feel, eat, behave, and live—to protect your body and your life. Consider this an opportunity to educate yourself about health care and be open to creating the necessary changes for improving your health. Have faith and be adaptable.

Tips For Setting New Priorities & Goals

1)   Structure your life and activities every day so that your health is top priority. Illness can be a reminder to slow down and take better care of yourself. Learn to set healthy limits with yourself and others.

2)   Say no when you feel uncomfortable saying yes. Let go of any guilt you may feel whenever you say no. People will respect you for setting and maintaining boundaries. And you'll be a good role model for them.

3)   Budget your time, energy, money, and activities wisely. Become efficient. Keep a "To Do" list. Do things on your list when you feel up to it. Ask for help when you need it. Give up feeling as if you have to do everything yourself. Let go of anything that is unnecessary, unimportant, or unhealthy to your body, psyche, or life.

4)   Plan your life according to your energy level. Slow down when your energy is low. When it increases, avoid the temptation to overexert yourself. It is important to nurture your energy and build up a reserve for healing (build it up as you would a savings account). Visualize any increase in your energy as a budding plant. Don't carelessly run over it with a plow. Nurture and feed it, and your energy will grow.

5)   Set new, realistic goals. Break them down into small, do-able steps so that your goals will not become a source of pressure. Take as much time as you need to accomplish your goals. Don't rush through life or follow anyone else's schedule. The fast lane is exciting, but it can be stressful and lead to illness. Have patience with yourself, especially when you are not feeling well. Always consider your health first.

6)   Surround yourself with supportive, happy, and loving people. Let go of those who cause you stress. Avoid negative people who drain you, such as unsupportive people who question the reality of your illness.

7)   Deal directly with any emotions associated with your illness—such as guilt, resentment, fear, disappointment, anger, rage, or insecurity.

8)   Develop a rock-solid foundation of unconditional self-love and acceptance. Remember that you deserve the same loving care as you give your family members, close friends, plants, and pets!

9)   Schedule time for being productive, time for relaxation, and time for exercise. And give yourself permission to have fun during the week. Enjoy creative projects or hobbies, go for walks and explore new places, listen to comedy, play a musical instrument, or plant some flowers.

10)   Make a list of your health care needs. Begin to schedule necessary appointments with your doctors, caregivers, and support people.

11)   Plan and prepare healthy meals. Learn to eat slowly; it helps with digestion and makes your food more pleasurable and satisfying.

12)   Get help with preparing meals. Many people enjoy cooking for others. Call local churches or organizations that may provide food programs.

13)   List things for which you are most grateful. Keep adding to the list.

14)   Meet with a friend once a week to share your desires, goals, and accomplishments. Reward each other with special acknowledgments.

15)   Make a "Treasure Map" of things that you want to create in your life. Cut out pictures from magazines or make drawings of what you desire, such as improved health, fitness, happiness, or a loving relationship. It is best to focus on one area of your life at a time. Make lists of what you want and what you don't want. Place the pictures and lists in a binder or make a collage for your wall. Review the pictures and lists each day. Believe in the possibility of creating the life you envision. (To order a *Life Treasure Map* kit, use the order form on page 233.)

Creating A Healthier Lifestyle

"Lifestyle" is defined as: "the consistent, integrated way of life of an individual as typified by his or her manner, attitudes, possessions, etc."
– *Webster's Unabridged Dictionary of American English,* Third College Edition, 1988

Dr. Leon Chaitow, author of *The Body/Mind Purification Program: How to be healthy in a polluted world* (A Fireside Book, published by Simon & Schuster, 1990), recommends a holistic plan for detoxifying and re-energizing your life. Specializing in osteopathy and natural therapies, Dr. Chaitow is the author of numerous books on health and nutrition. Whether it is work-related tension, chemical abuse, or environmental pollutants (from smog and cigarette smoke to harmful household products and unhealthy foods), the chances are you are feeling the effects of daily exposure to an increasingly toxic and stressful world. Fortunately, the marvelously resilient human body and mind can cope, with a little help from you. Dr. Chaitow recommends eating a detoxification diet for 10 or 30 days (ask your doctor or nutritionist for help). He also suggests that you do breathing exercises to calm tensions; do aerobics when you can to improve circulation and oxygenation; do stretching exercises to help eliminate wastes; practice meditation for coping in a stressful environment; get massages to help you relax your muscles and release toxins; use water therapies to detoxify and aid circulation; and do whatever else you can to stimulate healing and feel well.

Healthy Lifestyle Tips

16)   Make a list of lifestyle changes which may help you to feel better. Discuss the list with your doctor and begin to make those changes.

17)   Buy, grow, and eat organic foods. Whenever possible, avoid consuming foods treated with pesticides, waxes, fungicides, and sprays. Buy produce from farmers' markets or roadside stands. Eat healthy snacks. Carry a bottle of filtered water when you go out.

18)   Unless you have specific dietary requirements because of illness, you may benefit by eating more potatoes, grains, cereals, root and leafy vegetables, legumes, and fruits; and by eating less meats, fish, poultry, and dairy products. Meats, fish, poultry, and dairy products tend to have more pesticide residues; they are higher in fats, cholesterol, and calories; and they tend to be harder to digest. Producing meats and dairy products takes a toll on the environment.

19)   Each week get involved with creative projects (such as painting, playing an instrument, or gardening). Or, read about your creative interests. Talk with your family and friends about your hobbies. Share your artwork, music, or home-grown vegetables with your loved ones.

20)   Whenever possible, take quiet vacations, go on weekend trips, or do things that are fun and relaxing at home. Turn your home into a personal health club and spa. Set up a comfortable place where you can stretch or do light exercises. Have a friend give you a facial or give each other a massage. Convert your bathtub into a whirlpool. Make your home environment as comfortable as possible.

21)   Be aware of your energy level and your physical needs. Take breaks when necessary. Create more balance, harmony, and joy in your life.

22)   Create a pleasant, nurturing environment at home and at work.

23)   Simplify your life as much as possible.

24)   Have loving heart-to-heart talks with your family and friends.

25)   Spend more time in nature. Watch the stars. If you cannot leave home, read about exotic places or animals. Watch nature programs on TV.

26)   Schedule rest periods often. Make "siestas" part of your health care. (I often resisted taking naps in the afternoon because I felt as if I were missing out on doing something more fun. Yet now I appreciate my afternoon naps. It is a real luxury and a pleasant healing ritual.

Time & Life Management

27)   Focus on just one day at a time. Living in the present enhances your energy and power. Don't worry about the past or future. Learn from your past and make new plans for your future.

28)   Each morning, list what you must do during the day. Set up a simple schedule based on your list and energy level. Each night, review your list. What you did not complete during the day, add to a future list. Reward yourself for your accomplishments. If you have trouble remembering things, use notes, calendars, and lists. (This works!)

29)   Streamline your life by making more efficient use of your time. Being efficient is essential when living with illness and low energy. Conserve your time, money, and energy by using them wisely. Consolidate your trips and errands when you go out. Get help with errands and housework when necessary. If you need help, ask a social worker or your doctor for a referral to in-home services. Read *Too Busy To Clean? Over 500 Tips & Techniques To Make Housecleaning Easier* by Patti Barrett (New York: Wings Books, 1990).

30)   Alan Lakein, renowned time-management consultant and the author of *How To Get Control Of Your Time And Your Life*, writes: "...To waste your time is to waste your life, but to master your time is to master your life and make the most of it." He created a plan to help people determine the best use of their time and to gain control of their lives. He recommends working "smarter rather than harder." This allows you to do more of what you want, and helps you to enjoy life more.

31)   Rid yourself of material things that you no longer need or want. Sell or give away things you no longer use. Getting rid of clutter frees up your life and your mind. Clear out the old to bring in the new.

32)   Instead of driving all over town to shop or get information, use your telephone more. Many products can be ordered by phone and many stores have free delivery. Shopping at home—using mail order catalogs or computer networks—can save time, money, and energy.

33)   Use a calendar to keep track of your appointments and activities.

34)   Arrange with your bank to have your payroll, social security, or disability checks deposited directly into your account. Some banks give your credit for direct deposit. Arrange for your monthly bills (utilities, telephone, rent, or credit card accounts) to be automatically deducted from your account. Or, pay these bills over the phone.

35) Organize your life as much as possible. Begin with organizing your purse or wallet, desk, paperwork, files, bookshelves, personal records, bills, finances, property, etc. Begin organizing your work, household, health care plan, schedule, social and recreational activities.

36) Talk to friends, neighbors, or church members and develop a list of grocery stores and restaurants that will deliver groceries or meals to your home. More grocery stores are offering this service. Or find organizations that will donate food or meals to people who are ill.

37) Stephen R. Covey, author of *The 7 Habits Of Highly Effective People: Powerful Lessons in Personal Change* (Simon & Schuster, 1989), offers effective tips for getting organized in your work and personal life. He suggests that you create a personal vision—a mission statement to help you clarify all of your roles and goals. He offers a step-by-step pathway for solving personal and professional problems.

38) Schedule regular times to turn off your telephone in order to avoid disturbing your rest or sleep. Tell friends and family your schedule so they will call you only at appropriate times. Arrange for them to signal you if necessary. For example, they can ring once and call right back. Use an answering machine for messages or to screen your calls.

39)   Draw a pie chart to represent your life. Divide the chart into sections that represent time for health care, work, chores, quality time with family and friends, rest periods, entertainment, and exercise. How can you allot your time and energy more effectively? Draw this plan.

40)   Draw a bar chart that represents different aspects of your life. Give more height to areas that are working well and less height to areas that need more of your time and attention. Visualize, list, or chart ways to put your life into balance. Plan a new, fun, and healthful life.

Chapter 2. Promoting Physical Health

You may feel too ill or be unable to attempt any regular exercise. With some illnesses, such as Chronic Fatigue Syndrome, exercise may tend to aggravate symptoms. Still, most doctors recommend getting some form of exercise to maintain muscle tone, support general health, reduce stress and anxiety, and alleviate depression. The key is to pay attention to how you feel and to find an appropriate exercise. Light exercise (such as walking or stretching) may help you to feel better, both physically and mentally. Regular exercise can be good for your heart, circulation, nervous system, and immune system; and it also promotes sleep. Talk to your doctor about setting up a personal exercise plan.

Dean Ornish, M.D., author of *Dr. Dean Ornish's Program for Reversing Heart Disease* and *Eat More, Weigh Less*, has researched the value of proper exercise and diet. Since 1977 he has "directed landmark scientific research demonstrating that even heart disease can be reversed by changing diet and lifestyle, without drugs or surgery." During these studies, he and his colleagues made an unexpected and important discovery—that his program had dramatic effects on weight. They learned what motivates people to make and maintain comprehensive lifestyle changes over many years.

Patients in Dr. Ornish's study lost an average of twenty-two pounds during the first year, even though they were eating more food, and more frequently, than they had before the study. His approach is scientifically based on the *type* rather than the *amount* of food, creating a sense of abundance rather than deprivation. The meals are low in fat, allowing you to "eat more frequently, eat a greater quantity of food and still lose weight—simply, safely, and easily." Dr. Ornish has created a new approach to eating and living so that people can improve their health and well-being. They learn to heal emotional pain, loneliness, and isolation by providing nourishment for the body and soul.

According to Ann Cambra and Nancy Schluntz, authors of *Dieting: A Walk On The Light Side* (R&E Publishing, 1986): "...medical literature is in overwhelming agreement that regular exercise is beneficial to the functioning of your body as a whole, whether you lose weight or not. This is especially true after the age of thirty, when your body slows down of its own accord, as well as when your social/work habits fall into set patterns that demand less exertion of your body. Making healthier choices every day (regarding food, exercise, and lifestyle) can be a simple and an effective way to improve your well-being and your life."

The following tips offer ways to support your physical health. Discuss them with your doctor whenever necessary.

Self-Help & Healing Tips

41)   Nurture the healing force within you. Work with your inner physician (within your mind) to communicate with every cell in your body.

42)   Deal with your illness by facing it directly. Denying reality can cause negative consequences. Bernie Siegel, M.D. (who contributed material to the book *Chop Wood, Carry Water*) writes: "Accept your illness. Being resigned to an illness can be destructive and can allow the illness to run your life, but accepting it allows energy to be freed for other things in your life. See the illness as a source of growth.... View your illness as a positive redirection in your life...."

43)   Make peace with your illness. Fighting it causes stress and *dis*-ease.

44)   Keep a positive attitude. Accept limitations and focus on possibilities.

45)   Have faith that your health will improve. Have patience with yourself. Symptoms of chronic illness tend to wax and wane. Believe that you will feel better soon. And believe in your body's ability to heal itself.

46)   Nurture yourself by doing things that make you feel better.

47) Keep a daily journal of your healing and nurturing activities. Keep track of your thoughts, feelings, nutrition, goals, desires, and dreams. (To order a *Daily Health Care Workbook*, use the form on page 233.)

48) Schedule regular massages. Take time to relax in a bath or Jacuzzi.

49) Practice deep breathing and relaxation exercises regularly.

50) Take naps when needed. Get plenty of sleep during the night. If you have trouble sleeping, read a book or listen to relaxation tapes. Limit hearing bad news on late newscasts. Bad news can disturb your sleep.

51) Listen to uplifting music whenever you can. Sing and play a musical instrument when you are alone or with a loved one. Sing with a child.

52) Focus on the good things in your life. Make a list of things that you like about yourself. Stop comparing yourself to others who have more energy or better health. Why torment yourself if you don't have to?

Listening To Your Body

53) Pay attention to how your body feels. What is healing? What is not?

54)   Think loving thoughts about your body. Accept and love yourself.

55)   Make a list of the things that make you feel good. Include things that you enjoy doing and things that give you more energy.

56)   Eat only foods that agree with you or are healthy for you. Check with your doctor about having a food allergy test to rule out any food-related health problems. Studies have shown that many chronic illnesses have been linked to food allergies.

57)   Promote the healing power within your body. Visualize healing energy moving throughout areas where you feel pain, fatigue, or weakness.

58)   Develop a healing attitude. Say: "I am not a *victim* of illness. I can overcome adversity by taking responsibility for my body's needs."

59)   Practice deep breathing exercises to release tension, blocks, or negativity, and to promote healing. William Collinge, Ph.D., author of *Recovering From Chronic Fatigue Syndrome* (Putnam, 1993), writes: "You may choose to use the breath as the focus for your relaxation process. Take long, slow, and deep breaths into the belly. Concentrate on a particular aspect of the breath. Breath can be used in several ways. One way is to focus on the expansion and relaxation of your belly. Notice when you breathe in, the belly expands outward as the diaphragm moves down, making more room for the lungs. As you exhale, the belly is drawn back in. Follow the rhythm of this in-and-out movement, like a continuous circular motion or a wave. Another method is to count each in-breath and each out-breath, in pairs. Repeat this process up to ten. When you reach ten, begin again. Or focus on a sound or a word. Repeat the sound or word throughout the relaxation process. You can repeat a word on the out-breath or use a phrase such as, "I am healing now."

60)   Use "The Fifty-Percent Solution," as recommended by William Collinge, Ph.D., for conserving energy for healing. This plan has been effective for many of his patients who have serious illnesses and low energy. He states: "The essence of the fifty-percent solution is that you are spending half the energy you feel is available, and investing the other half in your body's healing process. It takes energy to heal. Energy that is spent outwardly is not available inwardly to energize your healing process. It takes self-discipline to hold back in this way. Recovery demands that you tune in to your body and truly respect the need to pace yourself."

61)   Bernie Siegel, M.D. believes that the body responds positively to self-love and peace of mind. The body gets "live" or "energy" messages when you say "I love myself." This is not the ego talking; it is self-esteem. It makes you feel that you are worthy. It helps you to believe in yourself and it tells you that you are of importance to the world. This attitude encourages your immune system to fight for your health.

Stress Reduction

Stress is a part of life that we all must learn to handle. Stressful thoughts can make us feel ill at ease—our stomachs cramp, palms sweat, mouths get dry, muscles contract, and our hearts quicken. Stress can make us tense, nervous, and anxious. It can cause high blood pressure, headaches, insomnia, stomach problems, or trigger life-threatening illnesses.

Virginia Wells, author of *50 All Natural Stress Busters* (Globe Communications, 1993) writes, "There are two important factors to consider about stress. First, it's the degree of stress you experience, coupled with your ability to handle it, that makes it either positive or negative. Second, YOU determine how stress affects you. Your habits, abilities and experience in handling stress, more than the nature of the stress itself, dictate that—which means that stress management is the key to emotional and physical health…. Our stress-response is our natural defense system at work—which means that, although we can't eliminate stress from our lives, we can learn to handle it better."

62) Herbert Benson, M.D. and Eileen M. Stuart, R.N., co-authors of *The Wellness Book: The Comprehensive Guide to Maintaining Health and Treating Stress-Related Illness* (Simon & Schuster, 1992), suggest a four-step approach to reducing stress. They call it: "Stop, Breathe, Reflect, and Choose." When you feel any stress, say "Stop" to yourself to interrupt the automatic stress response. Breathe deeply to release any physical tension and to initiate the relaxation response. Reflect on the problem and try to understand where the automatic response came from. Reflection is an effective tool to clarify the cause of your stress. Choose effective coping strategies to deal with stress.

63) Exercise or physical activity is an effective way to relieve stress, anger, or anxiety. If your energy is limited, try doing some light stretches in bed or while sitting in a chair. Or, try going for a walk or swim.

64) New research indicates that good nutrition can help your nervous system function better during times of stress. (*Delicious!* Nov., 1994).

65) Relax and listen to soft music while you take a soothing, warm bath.

66)   Limit or avoid drinking caffeinated beverages which can trigger stress and anxiety. Many herbal teas (such as chamomile, ginseng, cloves, lime or linden flowers, or peppermint) may help you to relax.

67)   Eating too much sugar can contribute to anxiety. It may deplete the body's B-complex and minerals which increases nervous tension, anxiety, irritability, and fatigue. Eat foods that have optimal nutritional value. Pay attention to how foods make you feel. Choose foods that have a calming effect.

68)   Avoid drinking alcohol or caffeine drinks, taking drugs, or smoking as a way of trying to reduce stress. These chemicals can throw your body's chemistry off-balance, causing more stress than relief.

69)   Avoid food additives such as monosodium glutamate (MSG), aspartame (sweetener), nitrates, and nitrites—which may produce allergic and anxiety symptoms, such as panic attacks, headaches, upset stomach, or dizziness. Dairy products are difficult for some people to digest; these foods may contribute to fatigue, depression, allergies, or anxiety. Avoid foods that are high in salt and fat because they may contribute to high blood pressure and heart problems.

70)   Talk to a dietitian or nutritionist about your vitamin and mineral requirements, and about foods/nutrients that relieve anxiety or stress.

71)   Loving thoughts and emotions will help to nurture your mind and body, and help to reduce stress. Say loving words to yourself. Release critical thoughts and images. Work with a psychotherapist, close friend, or support group to help you cope with fear, anger, and grief.

72)   Find a doctor who is trained in biofeedback. Ask your doctor to teach you how to use a biofeedback machine for stress reduction. Biofeedback is often helpful for: reducing blood pressure; decreasing tension, pain, and headaches; and promoting relaxation and sleep.

73)   Feel your emotions as much as possible. Cry if you need to; it releases pain and stress. Have "heart-to-heart" talks with loved ones or pets.

74)   Explore various stress-reduction techniques and regularly do the ones you enjoy. Try visualization exercises, reading, laughing, drawing, resting, listening to soft music, singing, or getting a massage or hug.

75)   Meditation is effective for reducing stress. Choose a technique that works best for you. Incorporate yoga into your relaxation program.

76) Jon Kabat-Zinn, Ph.D., author of *Full Catastrophe Living: Using the Wisdom of Your Body and Mind to Face Stress, Pain, and Illness* (Dell Publishing, 1990) and *Wherever You Go There You Are: Mindfulness Meditation in Everyday Life* (Hyperion, 1994) recommends a useful stress-reduction technique that he calls "body scanning." It is good for developing concentration and "flexibility of attention." To scan your body, focus on each area and linger there with your mind. Breathe in and out from each area a few times, then let go of it in your mind. Move your attention to the next area. Let go of any thoughts, images, tension, or fatigue with each out-breath. Breathe in energy, vitality, and relaxation. Begin body scanning by lying on your back, relaxing, and visualizing areas of your body. Start with your toes, feet, pelvis, torso, lower back, abdomen, upper back, chest, and shoulders. Feel any sensations as you go. Move to the fingers of both hands, up both arms, and return to your shoulders. Move your awareness through your neck, throat, face, and the back and top of your head. Breathe through an imaginary blow "hole" on top of your head. Breathe through your entire body, from the top of your head and out through your toes; then breathe in through your toes and out the top of your head. When you have completed the body scan, let yourself be silent and still. When you are ready, return your full attention to your body, and feel refreshed and rejuvenated.

Personal Care & Hygiene

77) Avoid exposure to germs whenever possible. Wash your hands frequently—especially during the flu season, after being out in public, or after handling money or playing cards. Don't allow people to cough at you. Give them a tissue if they need one. Or wear a protective mask if necessary. Avoid direct contact with the receiver on a public telephone or a drinking fountain. Use paper when sitting on a public toilet seat. While flushing a toilet, turn away from the forceful spray of the water to avoid germs.

78) Take good care of your teeth. See your dentist regularly to keep your teeth and gums healthy. Get a new toothbrush often. Use a natural, chemical-free toothpaste. Floss each day. If you have crowns or other dental work, you may want to use a strong floss that doesn't shred and one that moves easily between teeth (such as Glide™. For more information call, W. L. Gore & Associates, Inc. at 1-800-645-4337).

79) Soak your feet in warm water regularly (up to 15 minutes at a time). You may enjoy a vibrating foot-soaker. You can add oils or herbs to the water. After soaking, use a pumice stone or a loofa to smooth the bottoms of your feet. Massage your feet with your favorite lotion.

80) Take care of your skin (it is the body's largest organ). Find skin care products that are suitable for you. Choose natural, fragrance-free, chemical-free lotions. Health stores have a variety of natural products—such as brushes, loofas, and sponges (which help to remove dead skin cells and to stimulate circulation).

81) After you shower, use a natural, non-aluminum deodorant. One excellent deodorant is made of natural body crystals—formed of the mineral salt potassium alum. This product is hypoallergenic, fragrance-free, non-staining, economical, and environmentally safe.

Healthy Foods & Good Nutrition

82) Eat organically-grown foods to decrease your consumption of pesticides, chemicals, additives, and preservatives. Buy fresh, seasonal, locally-grown fruits and vegetables when possible. Choose a variety of whole, natural, unprocessed foods and healthy beverages.

83) Avoid or limit alcohol, caffeine, sodas, MSG, or anything that disagrees with you. Limit sugar and fat intake. Reduce yeast, wheat, dairy products, or other foods that may cause allergies.

84) Drink 8 glasses of purified, boiled, or spring water throughout each day. It is preferable to drink water at room temperature, rather than ice cold. Drinking water with meals may dilute the digestive juices.

85) Drink fruit juices sparingly as they are highly concentrated in fruit sugar. Or eat the raw, whole fruit instead to get more of the fiber.

86) Vitamin and mineral supplements and herbs should be taken only as recommended by your doctor, dietitian, or nutritionist to prevent any nutritional imbalances. Vitamin C, B vitamins, trace minerals, acidophilus, algae, digestive enzymes, wheat grass, flax seeds, flax seed oil, and/or aloe vera juice may be beneficial for dealing with chronic illness and for promoting general health.

87) Learn to prepare simple, low-calorie, low-fat, low-sugar, nutritious and delicious meals. Eat a variety of foods each day to get a balanced diet. Don't skip meals because it can slow down your metabolism.

88) Eat slowly while sitting down in a calm, stress-free environment. Listening to classical music may help you to enjoy your meal. Chewing your food well can help with digestion.

Weight Control

Consult your doctor before beginning any weight control program. Managing your weight is an important part of any health care plan. Being at your appropriate weight may help to prevent some health problems. If you are faced with chronic illness, you may have special dietary requirements. Consult a professional if chronic illness, medications, or treatments are causing you to gain or lose too much weight. There are hundreds of excellent health and nutrition books available. See "Recommended Reading" in this book or ask your doctor, a nutritionist, or dietitian for further information.

89)   Each day, make wise food choices. Eat a variety of foods to get adequate amounts of essential nutrients. You may wish to follow the "Food Guide Pyramid, A Guide To Daily Food Choices," developed by the U.S. Department of Agriculture and the U.S. Department of Health and Human Services. The guide suggests that you select about 6-11 servings from the bread, cereal, pasta, or rice group; 3-5 servings from the vegetable group; 2-4 servings from the fruit group, 2-3 servings from the milk, yogurt and cheese group; 2-3 servings from the meat, poultry, fish, dry beans, eggs and nuts group; and use fats, oils and sweets sparingly. If you have food allergies or cannot eat dairy, meat, or fish, modify this guide to meet your specific needs.

90)   If you want to lose weight and are having trouble doing so by yourself, join a support group or a weight management organization. Many hospitals, clinics, and schools have free or low-cost, effective programs for weight control and nutrition counseling/education. Many people have found organizations, such as Weight Watchers, to be beneficial, affordable, fun, and supportive. Some people prefer the structure of a group, while others find it restrictive. Discover what works for you.

91)   Join Overeaters Anonymous (O.A.), a 12-Step program that addresses physical, emotional, and spiritual hunger. People meet and share experiences in a safe and supportive environment. They help each other to follow 12 steps toward healing and encourage each other to recover from compulsive overeating and other unhealthy behaviors. A "sponsor" (a support person in "recovery") will offer you guidance.

92)   Keep a daily record of everything that you eat and drink. Records can give you a sense of control, help you remember what you have eaten, reinforce your weight goals, and help you plan a balanced diet.

93)   Try these weight control tips: Let yourself be the number one priority in your life. Exercise each day, even if it is just stretching and walking. Take a shopping list to the grocery store to prevent impulse buying.

94)   More weight control tips: Don't grocery shop when you are hungry; it can sabotage your efforts. Don't be obsessive about your weight. Don't eat too quickly. Don't eat when you're not hungry. Don't give your bathroom scale too much power over your moods or your life. (Many weight control counselors recommend not weighing yourself at all. Instead, they suggest focusing on healthy eating and proper exercise.)

95)   "The McDougall Plan" has helped many people to greatly improve their health. John A. McDougall, M.D. and Mary McDougall, authors of *The McDougall Program For Maximum Weight Loss* (Penguin Books, 1994), have created a simple, low-fat plan to help people effectively control their weight and lower their cholesterol.

96)   Develop your own plan for controlling your weight. Write what your goals are for a specific period of time. Create a realistic plan—one that responds to your needs. Keep track of your progress on charts or in a notebook. Find an enthusiastic support person and begin helping each other to achieve your goals. Give each other reward stickers.

97)   An important key to weight management and good nutrition is "portion control." If you keep food portions small, you may be able to continue eating the foods you enjoy. Focus on quality, not quantity.

98) Almost every weight control plan addresses the need for behavior modification. Here are some good examples: Don't eat while you're standing up. Sit down, relax, and eat slowly. Don't read or watch TV while eating. Focus on enjoying the taste and texture of your food.

99) Eat only when you are hungry; then stop eating before you feel full. Learn to say "No!" to foods that are unhealthy for you.

100) When you want to eat and you're not hungry, try writing down what role food plays in your life. Shift your focus away from food. Refocus your energy and attention to other things that give you pleasure. Keep a list of the things that you enjoy doing, besides eating.

101) Reward your successes for setting healthy limits with food and for achieving your goals. Set up a non-food reward system. For example, meet a friend and go for a walk instead of meeting for lunch.

102) Plan ahead—especially for the holidays, parties, or dining out. For potluck parties, consider taking healthy foods and beverages. Many low-calorie and low-fat entrees can be prepared in delicious ways so that everyone will enjoy them. You don't even have to tell people (especially your kids) that your delicious foods are low-cal and healthy!

103) Begin making healthy dietary changes. Repeat what works. If you backslide, don't feel badly. Just begin again. If you are offered food that you cannot eat, say "no thank you," without justifying your reply.

104) Limit the amount of tempting, high calorie snacks you keep at home.

105) Keep your favorite, healthy foods readily available.

106) Do not overeat when you feel ill, tired, or under stress. Delegate chores and errands. Rest whenever you need to.

107) Instead of turning to food to reduce anxiety, turn to other methods. Try deep breathing exercises, listening to soothing music, or walking.

108) If you overeat compulsively (or if you starve, binge, and purge), see a therapist who specializes in treating eating disorders or anxiety.

109) No amount of food can ever fill an emotional void or solve an emotional problem. Try to understand what might be motivating your overeating. Overeating can be a symptom of clinical depression. People often overeat when what they want is intimacy, love, support, or pleasure. Food, however, is no substitute for those feelings and desires.

Some people overeat when they feel angry, anxious, lonely, tired, or depressed. Deal directly with your emotions. Talk to a close friend.

110)   Set a realistic weight goal that you can maintain over time. Instead of dieting, develop healthy, low-fat eating habits for the rest of your life. Include plenty of fiber and water to help your digestion.

111)   Think positively when you see yourself in a mirror. Create positive mental images and thoughts about your body, weight, and health. During the day, and before you go to sleep each night, say loving, nurturing affirmations about your body. Keep a list of things that you like about your body. Louise L. Hay's book, *I Love My Body: A 30-day affirmation guide to a healthy, beautiful body* (Hay House, 1985) offers wonderful and supportive affirmations for your body and soul.

112)   Geneen Roth, author of *When Food Is Love: Exploring The Relationship Between Eating And Intimacy* (Plume, 1991) writes, "We live in a diet-obsessed culture. If you try to lose weight for others it may not work and you may end up gaining weight. Diets often lead to binges. Like yourself enough to take care of yourself. Some people overeat, then exercise to lose weight. It is best to exercise because you enjoy it. Listen to your body's needs." She suggests these tips:

Deeply explore one area of life to find answers to other areas. What you learn when you break free from obsession with food is what you need to learn about intimacy: commit yourself, tell the truth, trust yourself, know your pain will end, laugh easily, cry easily, have patience, and be willing to be vulnerable. Release your fears and anything else that causes you pain. Allow yourself to feel love.

113)   Believe in yourself and in your ability to control your weight. Visualize yourself at your goal weight; allow your mind to support your body.

Exercise

Ask your doctor about establishing a personalized exercise program that you can do while you are ill. Create a program that is appropriate for your energy level and any physical limitations. Almost anyone can do light stretching or walking. You may need to work with a physical therapist to rebuild muscle tone and strength. Combine walking, stretching, and low-impact aerobics if possible.

114)   Rebecca Eastman, author of *Full Circle Fitness*, believes that inactivity causes health risks, such as problems with the heart, body, and mental outlook. She says it increases your percentage of body fat and weakens the efficiency of your muscles, joints, and circulatory system. Inactivity speeds up the aging process and makes you vulnerable to disease, injury, and fatigue. It decreases your ability to concentrate and it can lower your self-esteem. However, regular exercise can help to remedy these problems. She defines four variables to consider for an appropriate exercise program: 1) Type (mode of exercise); 2) Duration (length of the workout); 3) Frequency (how often you work out); and 4) Intensity (how hard you work out).

115) Exercise of the appropriate type and duration is usually energizing, rather than fatiguing. Lack of oxygen can cause fatigue; exercising boosts your body's ability to take in oxygen and use it to make new energy, according to Dr. Robert Cooper, author of *Health & Fitness Excellence*. He writes: "Studies suggest that regular exercise can boost the body's resistance to a wide range of illnesses and diseases."

116) Make exercise fun. Many people enjoy swimming and walking, which are excellent, low-impact aerobic exercises. Walk where you can breathe fresh air and avoid fumes from traffic.

117) Walk on the beach to get fresh air and invigorating "negative ions."

118) Join a health club, if possible. Use the treadmill and Cybex® machines.

119)   Some exercise machines, such as Cybex, have been designed for people who are getting back into shape or for those recovering from illness or injury. Many health clubs have swimming pools, whirlpools, and saunas which can be healing and relaxing. Exercising in the pool is fun and less strenuous on the body.

120)   Whatever form of exercise you choose, listen to your body's needs and only move at your own pace. Take breaks when necessary.

121)   Dr. Neil Gordon, author of *Chronic Fatigue: Your Complete Exercise Guide*, writes: "Start your exercise program slowly and progress gradually, as your condition permits. Always include both a warm-up and a cool-down of at least five minutes' duration." Stretching is part of a good exercise program and it should always precede aerobic exercise. Stretching relaxes you mentally and physically. Try to do stretching and aerobics 3 to 5 times a week. Muscle-strengthening exercises can be added to your routine when you are ready. If illness has impaired your ability to function, use isometric muscle-strengthening before more strenuous exercises. (Isometric exercise involves tensing one set of muscles for a period of seconds, in opposition to another set of muscles or to an immovable object.) Exercise your options—choose exercises that are easy and enjoyable.

122)   Many fitness experts recommend walking as a primary fitness activity. Dr. Gordon writes, "Walking is one of the best ways to get moving down the road to optimal health."

123)   Exercise can often relieve discomfort and stress, both psychological and physical. For those with chronic illness, mild low-impact aerobic exercise (such as walking, swimming, or using a stationary bike) is usually recommended—rather than more strenuous activities.

124)   Keep a daily journal of your exercise efforts. Place reward stickers in your journal, next to your accomplishments. Or reward yourself with a warm bath after exercising to relax your mind and muscles.

125)   Exercise does not have to be complicated. In fact, you don't even have to leave home. You can work out while watching a low impact exercise video. Stretch, using exercise bands, or while you are doing chores or housework. Or play your favorite music and dance, if possible.

126)   Yoga is a healing exercise for many people who are ill. Many basic yoga movements are done on a mat. Slow, careful movements prevent exhaustion. Over time, yoga builds muscle tone, strength, and energy. Combined with meditation, it is a soothing and relaxing experience.

Physical & Movement Therapies

If you have been bedridden because of chronic illness and feel weak, talk to your doctor about getting physical or movement therapies. These rehabilitative therapies help to rebuild strength and muscle tone, and help to relieve chronic pain. Physical therapy is used to help relieve symptoms, prevent or correct deformities, and to improve body function. Specific techniques can be designed by a therapist to meet individual needs. A therapist begins treatment and then teaches you exercises to do on your own at home. Movement therapy can help you to preserve or increase your range of motion and to prevent muscle atrophy.

Physical therapy involves the alignment of the musculoskeletal framework and can be effective in the treatment of diseases affecting muscles and joints. A number of modalities are used—such as heat, massage, electrical stimulation, and manipulations. Among the advantages of physical therapy are: no drugs are used and surgery on joints can sometimes be avoided. You can also do some exercises at home to correct problems and strengthen muscles (Birkedahl, 149).

127)   Find a competent physical or movement therapist. Ask friends or your doctor for a referral. A therapist must be trained and licensed in order to practice. Be sure your therapist is fully licensed and qualified to administer therapy.

128)   If you must spend a lot of time in bed, you should be in a comfortable position, but not all curled up. It is best to use a firm mattress and a comfortable pillow that supports your neck. Ask your physical therapist or doctor about mild exercises that you can do in bed.

129)   In "passive" exercise, patient do nothing but relax. Heat applications may be used while a therapist moves their limbs. This helps prevent adhesions and muscle shortening; it is preliminary to active movement (Cooper, *Woman's Health & Medical Guide*).

130)   In "isometric" exercise, muscles are tensed but there is no motion of the joint. This can help to maintain strength and help with circulation. Breathe normally while doing these exercises. Here are two examples of isometric exercises which are often done several times a day after surgery: 1) Tighten your knee caps for a few seconds, then relax, and repeat several times; 2) While lying on your back, gently point and extend your toes down as far as possible and hold briefly. Then flex your toes toward you and hold briefly. Repeat these movements.

131)   In "resistive" therapy, the patient moves against weights or against the therapist. This strengthens specific muscle groups.

132)   Physical therapy can include the use of heat, cold, or massage. Heat application helps to reduce stiffness, increase circulation, and reduce muscle spasms. Heat can be soothing. Cold has anesthetic effects and relieves inflammation. Usually a 5-minute application is enough to provide relief. A massage warms your skin, stimulates nerve endings, relaxes muscles, and it can help rid your body of toxins.

133)   Splints can be used to limit movement if your joints are swollen and painful. In mild cases, an elastic bandage may provide enough support and protection. While a limb is splinted, isometric exercises can help to maintain strength.

134)   Consider myotherapy (muscle therapy), developed by Dr. Desmond Tivy. "Myotherapy is a safe, drug-free way to eliminate pain caused by stress, accidents, sports, disease, and job hazards," according to Bonnie Prudden in her book, *Myotherapy: Bonnie Prudden's Complete Guide to Pain-Free Living*. It is the foundation of her total program for lifelong fitness, health, and freedom from pain. She believes that you can learn to find and press your own "trigger points" for pain relief, and you can reeducate your muscles, and tone and stretch them to prevent pain.

Chapter 3. Holistic Health Care

Many people with chronic illness or pain benefit from holistic health care, or "alternative" forms of healing, which treat the "whole" person. Such therapies (including acupressure, acupuncture, biofeedback, chiropractic, herbal medicine, homeopathy, hypnosis, massage, meditation, naturopathy) can enhance health, reduce stress, increase energy, and promote an overall sense of well-being.

Corey Weinstein, M.D., a San Francisco-based physician and author, writes: "Natural medicine refers to those techniques and skills, or adjustments in living habits, which help and encourage the individual to reach a better state of health through internal healing mechanisms. All biological systems have the capacity for self-organization and renewal. The human body has an inherent power to heal itself. Natural therapies try to stimulate the body/mind's internal mechanisms to restore healthy structure and function."

According to Dr. Weinstein, "Natural medicine depends on one's own healing effort. Great attention is placed on self-care. Proper food, rest, fresh air, and appropriate exercise are as important as any medicine, herb, or treatment. Natural treatment implies respect for the human body and its ways of overcoming illness. By understanding their own rhythms and healing processes, most people will learn to find the time and support required for healing."

Natural medicine views illness as an individual expression of imbalance. Symptoms are seen as evidence of disharmony. They are an attempt to restore order to the body. Symptoms are analyzed to track the progress of treatment. Diagnosis is viewed as the understanding of the phenomenon of illness. The whole person is taken into account. Treatment is individualized and based on the entire expression of a disorder. Self-care (what the client does) is emphasized.

Excellent resources on this topic include: *Alternative Medicine: The Definitive Guide*, compiled by The Burton Goldberg Group (Puyallup, WA: Future Medicine Publishing, 1993); the *Alternative Medicine Yellow Pages: The comprehensive guide to the new world of health*, compiled and edited by Melinda Bonk (Future Medicine Publishing, 1994); *Alternative Medicine: Natural Home Remedies* (a booklet and video tape by Future Medicine Publishing, 1994); and *Alternative Medicine Digest* (a bi-monthly journal that reports the best, the boldest, and the newest information from the field of holistic health). Call: 1-800-720-6363.

You may wish to explore several holistic health care options for your own healing program. Following is a brief overview of some of these therapies and techniques.

Holistic Therapies & Techniques

135)   **Acupuncture** was developed in China over 5,000 years ago. The Chinese believe that health requires a balanced flow of Qi (or Chi), vital life energy present in all living organisms. Qi moves in the body along twelve energy pathways or "meridians." These pathways are linked to specific organs and organ systems. Points in the body are stimulated to enhance the flow of Qi by inserting special needles into these points, just under the skin. This helps to correct and rebalance the flow of Qi, allows energy to flow freely, and helps to relieve pain and restore health. (The Burton Goldberg Group. *Alternative Medicine.* 1993, 37-46.) Acupuncture can help to increase the immune response by balancing the flow of life energy throughout the body. This complete system of healing provides effective treatment for a wide range of conditions—such as colds, flu, addictions, and chronic fatigue. It may be effective as an adjunctive treatment for AIDS.

136)   **Acupressure** is similar to acupuncture, except that needles are not used, according to J. V. Cerney, D.C., author of *Acupuncture Without Needles* (Parker Publishing, 1983). Specific acupressure techniques (applying pressure with the fingers, thumbs, fists, or palms) are used to relieve pain, discomfort, and tension in the body. Acupressure can be helpful in the treatment of numerous ailments—such as fatigue, migraines, colds, tension, hearing and eye problems, blood pressure problems, asthma, arthritis, and pain.

137) **Aromatherapy**, a branch of herbal medicine, uses the medicinal properties found in the essential oils of various plants. The oil or "essence" of a plant is extracted from its flowers, leaves, branches, or roots. When the oils are absorbed by the body's tissues, they may have a therapeutic effect. Inhaling the fragrance of certain essential oils can have a stimulating or a calming effect. Plants and essential oils have been used for healing since ancient times—in Egypt, Italy, India, China, and other countries. Today these oils are used in products such as antiseptic creams, skin ointments, and liniments for arthritic pain. Aromatherapy has become more popular in the United States because of consumer demand for nontoxic and nonthreatening restorative therapies. (The Burton Goldberg Group, 53) Health food stores carry essential oils and aromatherapy kits.

138) **Biofeedback** training helps people learn to change and control their body's vital functions to improve their health. Using a simple electronic device, one learns to consciously regulate normally unconscious bodily functions—such as breathing, heart rate, and blood pressure. Biofeedback can help to reduce stress, eliminate headaches, control asthma, restore injured muscles, and relieve pain. Electrodes are placed on the skin as a person uses relaxation, meditation, or visualization techniques to achieve a desired result (such as relaxing muscles or lowering blood pressure, heart rate, or temperature). A practitioner monitors changes in bodily functions, including skin temperature and electrical conductivity of the skin. Muscle tension is observed with an electromyogram, heart rate is monitored with an electrocardiogram, and brain waves are recorded with an electroencephalogram. (The Burton Goldberg Group, 73-79)

139) **Bodywork** therapies (massage, deep tissue manipulation, movement awareness, and energy balancing) can improve the structure and functioning of the body. Bodywork can help reduce pain, soothe injured muscles, stimulate circulation, and promote deep relaxation. It is important to maintain an awareness of your body and to take care of it. Staying aware of your body can help you to feel more alive, conscious, and whole. One way to achieve this awareness is through touch. When touch is given with love and care, healing can take place. Some types of bodywork (such as Rolfing or Trager) help release "body memories" of previous pain/trauma stored in the body.

140) **Chiropractic** treatment involves adjusting the spine and joints and can influence the body's nervous system and natural defense mechanisms to alleviate pain and improve health. Qualified chiropractors can effectively treat back problems, headaches, injuries, and traumas. Chiropractors must have four years of chiropractic college, plus two years of pre-chiropractic education. Students must pass a state chiropractic board examination and complete 600 hours of training before receiving a license. Chiropractors must study biochemistry to understand the application of foods and supplements in the treatment of disease. Advantages of this treatment include: some insurance companies cover it; no drugs are used; and the use of nutrition, exercise, and sensible practices of living helps you maintain an active part in your own health management (Birkedahl, 144-145).

141) Martin Borge, D. C., in Marin County, California, states, "Joint pain, muscle stiffness, and back or neck problems can drain your body's energy for healing. Your body needs energy to compensate for any misalignment or pain. Poor posture and back pain, in general, may make you more susceptible to chronic fatigue and illness. A qualified, holistic chiropractor may help you relieve such problems. The holistic approach addresses the cause of any misalignment, not just the symptom. Underlying causes may include: nutritional deficiencies, allergies, emotional or psychological stress, or unhealthy lifestyle choices. Not getting enough sleep can perpetuate muscle or skeletal problems. Drinking too much coffee or alcohol can overtax the kidneys, liver, and adrenal glands, interfering with proper immune function. A weakened adrenal system can cause more susceptibility to allergies, fatigue, and illness. You may consider a 'non-force,' gentle technique if you are uncomfortable with traditional chiropractic techniques."

142)   **Environmental Medicine** explores the role of dietary and environmental allergens in health and illness. (The Burton Goldberg Group, 205-213) Exposure to chemicals, dust, mold, pollen, and certain foods may cause allergic reactions that can dramatically influence diseases—such as asthma, hay fever, headaches, or depression. Specialists in this field are helping patients with chronic illness to explore ways to improve their health. Causes of environmental sensitivities include: heredity/genetics, poor nutrition, infection, chemical exposure, and stress. Tests for environmental illness include: the elimination diet (avoiding certain foods); skin testing (to detect any allergic reactions to pollen, molds, and foods); injecting small amounts of allergenic material just beneath the skin; Radio Allergo Sorbent Test (RAST), a blood test to diagnose allergies; and a thyroid function test. An overactive or underactive thyroid can result in increased allergies, skin problems, fatigue, nervousness, gastrointestinal problems, sleep disturbance, weight problems, swelling, and pain. Increased use of chemicals and medications complicates the treatment of various illnesses. Effective treatment must involve cooperation of the patient, who may need to make changes in his or her diet, lifestyle, and environment.

143) **Enzyme Therapy** involves using plant and pancreatic enzymes to restore health by improving the digestion and absorption of essential nutrients. Treatment includes enzyme supplements, a healthy diet, and whole foods. Plant enzymes enhance the body's vitality by strengthening the digestive system. Pancreatic enzymes are beneficial to the digestive system and the immune system. As proper digestive functioning is restored, many acute and chronic conditions may be remedied. (The Burton Goldberg Group, 215-223)

144) **Guided Imagery** (or visualization) involves using the mind to evoke a positive physical response. The technique, in a relaxed state of mind, can reduce stress, slow heart rate, stimulate the immune system, and reduce pain. Imagery has three characteristics that make it beneficial for healing: 1) It directly affects physiology; 2) Through mental processes of association and "synthesis," it provides insight into one's health; and 3) It has an intimate relationship with emotions, which are often at the root of many health conditions. (The Burton Goldberg Group, 244-252) In a relaxed state, try visualizing your immune system getting rid of the viruses, bacteria, or toxins that may be causing your illness. Then, visualize yourself as healthy.

145)   **Herbal Medicine** has been used in all cultures throughout history. Healers, pharmacists, and physicians have dried plants for use as medicines. Today numerous prescription drugs are derived from trees, shrubs, or herbs. Some are made from plant extracts; others are synthesized to mimic natural plant compounds. Scientific documentation now exists regarding use of herbs for health conditions, including premenstrual syndrome, indigestion, insomnia, heart disease, cancer, and HIV. (The Burton Goldberg Group, 253-271)

146)   **Homeopathy** involves treating patients by using minute, nontoxic doses of plant, mineral, or animal substances. Specific medicines are chosen based upon the "Law of Similars." This law "formulates the parallel action or similarity between the toxic potential of a substance and its therapeutic action." (Horvilleur, 8-9) Homeopathic remedies stimulate the natural defenses of the body in order to make them more effective; they work with the body rather than against it.

Symptoms are the body's efforts to deal with stress and to defend or heal itself. Homeopathic medicines provide a gentle but powerful healing stimulus. ("Discover Homeopathy," a catalog by Homeopathic Ed. Services. Call: 1-800-359-9051 for information, books, or tapes.)

147) **Hydrotherapy**, used for thousands of years by many cultures, involves the use of water, ice, steam, and hot and cold temperatures for healing and maintaining health. Treatments include: immersion of the body in water; use of a steam bath, sauna, or sitz bath; colonic irrigation; or hot and cold compresses. Hot water can stimulate immunity, and soothe and relax the body. Cold water can tone muscles and reduce fever. Alternating hot and cold water can stimulate adrenal and endocrine glands, reduce congestion, alleviate inflammation, and activate organ function. (The Burton Goldberg Group, 281)

148) **Hypnotherapy** is used to manage a wide range of medical and psychological problems. Hypnosis and self-hypnosis can help people reduce pain; lose weight; stop smoking; reduce stress or anxiety; overcome fears, phobias, or depression; recover from trauma; or stop alcohol and drug abuse. It can also help people to increase self-esteem and build physical strength. Some advantages are: no drugs are used (sometimes it can take the place of pain-killing or tranquilizing drugs);

and it is safe (no one can make you do anything that you do not want to do). While hypnotherapy may not be for everyone, it has become more acceptable in the medical community. (Birkedahl, 146)

149)   Marilyn Gordon, certified hypnotherapist and author of *Healing Is Remembering Who You Are* (Robert D. Reed Publishers, 1995), teaches readers and workshop participants to find their powerful healing essence within. Her practical, inspirational, and easy-to-use book provides specific hypnotherapy techniques and self-healing processes. She reveals fascinating stories about actual hypnotherapy experiences (such as healing food or eating disorders; healing attitudes; dealing with feelings of abandonment, unworthiness, intimidation, or loneliness; healing sexual abuse; and recovering from other problems).

150)   **Light & Colored Light Therapy** are being studied in major hospitals and research facilities throughout the world. Results show that full-spectrum, ultraviolet, colored, and laser light can help to reduce chronic pain, stress, and depression; as well as help treat immune disorders and sleep problems. The body's internal "clock" (which controls sleep, hormone production, body temperature, etc.) can be thrown off balance under certain conditions, such as a lack of light, "seasonal affective disorder" (S.A.D.) or the "winter blues."

Sunlight and other forms of light therapy can readjust the body's natural rhythm and treat related health problems. Some studies show that different colors of light have different effects on the body. Bright light and colored lights may alter neurochemical production in the brain, stimulate the nervous system, inhibit or stimulate hormone production, reduce stress and pain, and induce relaxation. Light rays strike the retina of the eye and are converted into nerve currents. John Downing, O.D., Ph.D., Director of the Light Therapy Department at the Preventive Medical Center of Marin in San Rafael, CA, found that a deficiency of light caused diminished brain function, including learning disabilities, poor concentration, mental fogginess, poor memory, fatigue, and mood swings. Light therapy can significantly reduce or eliminate these symptoms. (The Burton Goldberg Group, 319-329)

151)   **Massage** may be the oldest and simplest of medical treatments. For thousands of years, some form of massage or laying on of hands has been used to heal and soothe people who are ill or stressed. Today there is overwhelming scientific evidence that confirms the benefits of massage. There are many types of massage and bodywork; some treat physical needs, while others delve into psychological and spiritual aspects. Massage can relax the body and mind; improve

circulation; increase energy; reduce muscle pain; and improve posture, flexibility, and muscle tone. Massage can help relieve congestion. It can act as a "mechanical cleanser," stimulating lymph circulation, hastening elimination of wastes and toxins, and enhancing immunity. Massage can relax muscle spasms and relieve tension. By helping to improve circulation and ease strain on the heart, it can help to compensate for lack of exercise and muscular contraction in people who are inactive because of injury, illness, or age.

152) The Alexander Technique was developed by Frederick M. Alexander to correct faulty posture in daily activities that cause serious physical and emotional problems. This simple and effective approach rebalances the body through awareness, movement, and touch.

153) The Feldenkrais Method was developed by Moshe Feldenkrais, who based it on his experience with martial arts, physiology, anatomy, psychology, and neurology. Our "self-image" is central to the theory, since we speak, move, think, and feel according to self-image. To change our body movements, we must change that image. This method helps people to move more easily. It is useful for those with limitations of movement caused by stress, accidents, back problems, or illness.

154)   Reflexology deals with specific reflex areas in the hands or feet that correspond to organs, glands, or other parts of the body. Appropriate reflex areas are stimulated, and the organ, gland, or body is relieved of stress or tension. This can promote relaxation, improve circulation, and unblock nerve impulses to restore the body's balance.

155)   Rolfing, developed by biochemist Ida P. Rolf, Ph.D., is based on the idea that human function is improved as parts of the body (head, torso, pelvis, legs, and feet) are properly aligned. Dr. Rolf believed that balance and poise could be reestablished by manually manipulating and stretching the body.

156)   Shiatsu means "finger pressure" in Japanese. It is a system of healing that balances the body's energy field (or Qi/Chi). Specific pressure points are massaged to ease aches, pains, tension, and fatigue. Shiatsu is an effective preventive therapy and it helps to revitalize the person.

157)   Swedish Massage involves systematically stroking, kneading, and pressing soft tissues of the body to improve the body's fluid balance. Oil may be used as muscles, ligaments, and tendons are massaged. Strokes are long and smooth, deep or soft, depending on one's needs.

158)   Therapeutic Touch™ was developed by Dolores Krieger, Ph.D., R.N. and Dora Kunz. Generally, there is no physical contact between patient and practitioner. A therapist's hands are 2" to 6" away from blockages in the patient's energy field to revitalize energy flow where necessary, to release congestion, or to remove obstructions. Effective in treating various medical conditions, it can help decrease anxiety, reduce pain, and ease problems of the autonomic nervous system. Hands-on touching is used when treating a fracture or other injury.

159)   The Trager Approach, developed by Milton Trager, M.D., involves intuition and movement reeducation. (The Burton Goldberg Group, 106) Gentle, rhythmical touch is combined with movement exercises. Clients learn to recognize and release habitual patterns of tension, present in posture and movement. No specific techniques of movement or massage are used. The practitioner feels how the client is holding his or her body and applies rocking, pulling, and rotational movements to the client's head, torso, and appendages to gently loosen tense muscles and stiff joints. This approach helps people who suffer from neuromuscular disturbances—caused by injury, disease, or aging.

160) **Meditation** is a safe and simple way to balance and rejuvenate physical, emotional, and mental states. Many people find it effective for reducing stress and pain; others incorporate it into an overall treatment for various conditions or illnesses; and many use it to maintain high-level wellness. Studies now confirm its clinical effects on health. Meditation may help to enhance immune function; reduce depression and anxiety; and promote physiological, psychological, and spiritual well-being. As life becomes more complex and stressful, it is essential to take time to quiet the mind and relax the body.

161) Meditation can involve focusing your attention on your breath, an image, or a sound (called a "mantra") to still your mind and create greater awareness and clarity. Or meditation can involve "mindfulness"—sitting quietly and observing thoughts, feelings, and senses without reacting to them. Meditation can be easy to learn and use. It can be practiced at home, in an office, in the hospital, or while walking or sitting in a natural setting.

162) Meditation can be healing to your body, mind, and spirit. The daily practice of meditation can be one of the most effective means of promoting your health and immunity—while reducing stress, frustration, and fatigue.

163) Try a variety of meditation techniques and find one that you enjoy. Some methods are more "active," such as visualization techniques or listening to meditation tapes, which lead you through a relaxation process. Another active technique involves mental alertness and experiencing your Higher Power. More "passive" forms of meditation clear your mind of most thoughts for deep relaxation. Listening to a meditation tape before you sleep might help you relax and sleep better.

164) Sit comfortably in a chair. Take a few deep breaths. Close your eyes. Visualize your immune system functioning normally. Visualize your white cells healing your body and imagine your body becoming stronger. Take time to assimilate and enjoy this healing experience.

165) **Naturopathy** deals with underlying causes of disease, such as ridding the body of toxins and waste. A naturopathic doctor develops a treatment program by taking into account a client's history, lifestyle, and work. Various holistic therapies may be used, including acupuncture, counseling, herbal medicine, homeopathy, and nutrition. A client is taught to follow a cleansing, high-fiber, and low-fat diet. Often a vegetarian diet is recommended. Appropriate vitamin and mineral supplements and herbs may be recommended to help counteract the effects of long-term, unhealthy eating habits. No drugs are used. Talk with your primary care doctor before agreeing to any treatment; and find a qualified practitioner. For more information, read *Encyclopedia of Natural Medicine* by Michael Murray, N.D. and Joseph Pizzorno, N.D. (Rocklin, CA: Prima Publishing, 1991).

166) **Qi Gong / Chi Kung** (pronounced "cheekung") is an ancient Chinese system of simple movement, breathwork, and meditation. By learning to do Qi Gong, you can strengthen, cleanse, and circulate your body's vital energy (Qi). Life energy ("bioelectricity") is called "Qi" or "Chi" by the Chinese, "Ki" by the Japanese, and "Prana" by Yogis. It is known to be effective in the prevention and treatment of a wide range of chronic and degenerative diseases. Using this energy for healing can help to restore vitality and physical health, increase energy and strength, encourage restful sleep, stimulate the immune system, relax and energize breathing, improve digestion, relieve stress-related illness, and encourage longevity. Qi Gong techniques can enhance the process of self-healing and support the maintenance of optimum health. The gentle mind-body exercises require little physical effort, and they are easy to learn and use. No equipment is needed.

167) "Traditional Chinese medicine developed out of the experiences accumulated over thousands of years in the battle against disease," according to Dr. Wu Chengde, of the Houston Institute of Chinese Martial Arts and Medicine. "It has helped more than a billion Chinese to both maintain their health and prevent illness. Qi Gong massage [using Qi energy] has a long history, and it has been an important part of Chinese medicine." Considered an effective method for treating and preventing disease, Qi Gong emphasizes smooth circulation of Qi, its proper level, and the quality of its circulation for health. Combined with Chinese herbs and acupuncture, it provides an effective treatment program. It is best to practice Qi Gong on a regular basis, whether alone or in a group. Dr. Chengde believes, "Chinese medicine is a treasure to human health and happiness." After moving to the U.S., he was surprised to discover that while many Americans enjoy Chinese food, they are not familiar with Chinese medicine and its achievements. He says, "Chinese medicine in America is still in its infancy." Cultural differences between the East and West can create misunderstandings about the concept and benefits of Qi.

168) Dr. Yang Jwing-Ming, author of *Chinese Qi Gong Massage* (YMAA Publ.,1992), writes: "Qi Gong massage regulates the Qi and blood circulating in the body, returning the body to its normal, healthy state. Modern Western medicine has given us healthier and longer lives but there are still many problems it cannot solve. Some treatments focus on providing relief from symptoms, rather than identifying and treating the root of the problem." Certain massage techniques can maintain health, help to slow the aging process, and improve health and well-being. Relaxation massage increases the circulation of Qi and blood in particular areas or in the entire body, removing blockages or stagnation of Qi caused by exercising or aging.

169) Mantak Chia, author of *Chi Self-Massage: The Taoist Way of Rejuvenation* (Healing Tao Books, 1986), suggests a daily practice, including some of the following exercises. 1) Warm up in the morning. Open your heart first before you open your eyes. When you wake up, do not jump out of bed and do not open your eyes. Take your time before getting up. Have a good morning warm up and the whole day will run smoothly. 2) Check your energy level. With your eyes closed, put your palm on the navel area. Women, put the left palm over the navel and the right palm on top. Men, put the right palm on the navel with the left palm over it. Concentrate on your navel until you feel it become warm. 3) Start with the "inner" smile. If you can, get in touch with your inner smile; feel the flow of it; and guide the smile all the way down from the face to the neck and through the heart, lungs, liver, kidneys, pancreas, spleen, and sex organs. Smile into the digestive system and then the nervous system and spinal cord.

Smile to them and sense when the smile can get through. Keep smiling until pain or tension go away. 4) Smile through your organs. Take a little more time to smile through any obstructions. Concentrate your awareness by smiling to any place where there is a blockage, until it begins to clear. Disease always begins with a blockage of energy flow to an organ, gland, or major pathway. When energy is blocked from flowing through a major organ or gland, the organ or gland gets less energy, less blood flow, and less nutrition. Over time, the organ or gland will work less effectively. To keep healthy: eliminate tension, worry, and toxins each day so they do not accumulate in the body.

170)   **Qi Gong/Chi Kung Self-Massage Techniques** involve massaging points used in acupressure on your body to increase and balance your energy for healing. Learn Qi Gong and Qi Gong self-massage by taking a class from someone who is trained in this field. Or watch video tapes, listen to audio tapes*, or read books to learn basic techniques. It helps to observe the techniques being done or to see illustrations. Most of the techniques can be done lying in bed or sitting in a chair.

* Two audio tapes (Qi Gong Meditation by Beth Quist and Taoist Healing Imagery by Kenneth Cohen) are available from: Sounds True Recording, 735 Walnut Street, Boulder, CO 80302. (800) 333-9185.

171)   The following are some basic Qi Gong self-massages for the face, head, neck, and body. They are designed to relax you, restore energy, relieve stress or headaches, and reduce sinus congestion. Do them in any order at one time, or do a few at a time during the day. Do fewer massages well rather than more poorly. Breathe gently and deeply, use focused concentration and be aware of your breathing while doing Qi Gong. If you are ill, it may take a few weeks before you begin to experience results. Since the effects are subtle, have patience with yourself. Do a series of 9 of each of the exercises. It is best to do them 4 times, for a total of 36 if you can. If you cannot do all 36, do 9 or multiples of 9. (Thanks to Ellen Raskin for teaching me the following techniques.) Note: To begin, rub clean hands together to warm them.

-   **Rub Nose**. With the tips of your middle fingers, slowly rub the sides of your nose from the base at nostrils to the bridge between your eyes. Apply light pressure on upward movements and firmer pressure moving downward.

-   **Wash Face**. Place your fingertips at your jaw line. Stroking upward with your fingertips and hands, begin to make circles on each side of your face. Move your hands from chin to forehead. Continue down both sides of your face, along the hairline and then down to the chin.

- **Wipe Head**. Place your fingertips on your scalp above the forehead at hairline and stroke back over entire scalp ending at nape of neck. Begin again at sides of the hairline and stroke back to nape of neck.

- **Move Eyes**. Rub your hands together briskly to warm palms. Close your eyes and place the soft part of palm lightly against eyelids to apply slight pressure. Rotate eyes in circles 9 times in each direction. Move eyes in straight line from left to right 9 times and up and down 9 times. Remove your hands from your eyes and focus on a point in the distance and count to 9.

- **Scissor Rub**. Form a "v" with each hand—by holding your thumb and index finger together and also holding your remaining fingers together. Move your hands up to your ears so that your ears are inside the "v" (with thumb and index finger in back of ear and the rest of your fingers in front). Rub your hands down and close fingers, and then move your hands up again with fingers (in "v") spread open.

- **Rub Ears**. Rubbing the ears can help to balance the immune system and nervous system. Here are 3 self-massages for the outer ear. 1) Reach over your head with your right arm and grasp the top part of your left ear. Gently pull your ear upward 9 times. Repeat with left arm, gently pulling right ear upward 9 times. 2) Grasp upper, middle part of ear with thumb behind and index finger in front of ear. Pull out with a slight tug and rub 9 times. 3) Gently grasp both ear lobes in the same manner—pull down with a slight tug and rub 9 times.

- **Rub Neck**. Here are 2 neck exercises. 1) Back of the neck. Grasp one hand over the other behind your neck. Rub the back of your neck, as though you are pulling a towel back and forth it. Do 9 or 18. Reverse hands; repeat back and forth motion 9 or 18 times. 2) Massage throat by placing one palm under the front of neck, lightly holding your jaw. Alternate stroking right and left hands down the front of your neck to mid-chest. When moving down to the middle of your chest, raise your other hand; begin stroking down front of your neck. Do 9 or 18.

- **Grasp Fist**. Raise your arms in front of your body, hands forward and elbows slightly bent. Squeeze your hands into tight fists, placing the thumb on the outside. Then stretch out your fingers, as if pushing air away, relaxing so they become soft. Squeeze again. Repeat cycle.

- **Knead Belly**. This is considered one of the most important Qi Gong self-massage techniques, as it is the major center of your strongest reservoir of Qi energy. Place one flat hand over the other on your belly at the navel. Apply slight pressure to contact abdominal muscles. Using both hands together begin in small circular motions and slowly widen circles. Women rub to their left 18 times. Reverse hands, placing top hand on bottom and bottom hand on top. Now reverse direction and do the circular motions for 18 times. Men rub to their right for 18 times, then reverse hands and rub to their left for 18 times.

- **Sweep Arms**. Place one palm at the inner side of your upper arm. Sweep down length of arm to fingertips. Continue around the fingertips to front of hand, up the arm, and around to the shoulder. Repeat 9 or 18 times, then sweep your other hand in the same manner for 9 or 18 times.

- **Sweep Legs**. Sit down. 1) Place both palms on the inner sides of the ankle bones. Sweep both hands up your inner legs to your thighs. Repeat by placing your hands back at the ankles and sweep up with your palms. Always sweep from the ankle up. Do not go backwards. 2) Place both palms on your outer thighs. Sweep down to your outer ankle bones. Repeat by placing hands back on your thighs and sweeping down your outer legs. Note: Be sure to sweep up the inner leg and sweep down the outer leg.

- **Rub Balls of Feet**. Sit down on the floor. Grasp both feet by placing thumbs in the middle, under the balls of your feet. Rub until those spots are warm.

172)   **Sound Therapy** can be used for healing in a variety of ways. "Modern science has proven that sound influences your immune system, your pulse, your muscle control, and your emotions," states Linda Holloway (a renowned music therapist with degrees in music education, music therapy, and humanities). She presents music healing workshops for Unity centers. Her audio tape, "Feeling Better/Feeling Sound: How Sound Can Heal and Harmonize Your Life," is available through Unity Village, MO 64065. Her tape teaches ways to put the healing power of sound and music to work in your life and environment. She explores the role of sound in ancient and modern cultures and she provides scientific data on the effects of sound on the body and mind.

173)   **Yoga**, a gentle exercise, can be modified for people with chronic illness. Lorna Bell, R.N. and Eudora Seyfer co-wrote *Gentle Yoga: A Guide to Gentle Exercise* (Berkeley, CA: Celestial Arts, 1987) specifically for people with arthritis, stroke damage, multiple sclerosis, for those in wheelchairs, and for anyone who needs a gentle exercise. They write: "Yoga is a lifestyle. It's a non-competitive system for the development

of human potential and is based on the concept of self-worth. Yoga develops a feeling of individuality. No matter what your physical condition, your age, your abilities or disabilities, yoga uses what you have, recognizes the wonder of you, and makes you better...." There are many branches of yoga, but "hatha yoga" is the most popular in the U.S. Hatha yoga means "a balanced union—a system for creating the balanced well-being of the total person." The authors state, "Yoga joins body, mind, and spirit into a balanced whole. Postures and poses are combined with deep breathing, relaxation, a healthful diet, and proper thinking." Your body responds to deep breathing and stretching. As yoga's cleansing action begins to rid your body of toxins, you begin to feel better. Yoga is a slow, thoughtful system of stretching and balancing. One pose affects every muscle in the body. Poses activate and stimulate circulation, digestion, elimination, the nervous system, and the endocrine system. Yoga is a potent natural medicine with a preventive, holistic approach. You can experience deep relaxation, a calm mind, slower pulse, and brings the body to a state more receptive for healing. Yoga is not a religion. It is a whole system for improving life—for changing people, physically and mentally.

Chapter 4. Environmental Health

With an increase in the use and development of hazardous chemicals in our environment, it is essential to make every effort to ensure that our homes and offices are safe. Most of us are exposed every day to toxins that have been linked by researchers to headaches, illness, fatigue, depression, sterility, cancer, and birth defects. Many homes and office buildings contain substances that may be causing people to experience irritation, stress, allergies, and environmental illness. Through education, awareness, and effort, we must reduce pollution. Read this excellent resource book: *Sinus Survival: A Self-Help Guide for Allergies, Bronchitis, Colds, and Sinusitis* by Dr. Robert S. Ivker (New York: Putnam, 1992).

Reduce Toxins At Home & At Work

174)   Read books on how to detoxify your home and office to protect yourself and your family from health hazards. Excellent resources are: *The Nontoxic Home & Office* (Jeremy P. Tarcher, 1992) by author and consumer advocate, D. L. Dadd; *Healthy Homes in a Toxic World* by M. M. Breecher, and S. Linde (John Wiley & Sons, 1992); and/or *Your Home, Your Health, & Well-Being* by D. Rousseau, W. J. Rea, and J. Enwright (Ten Speed Press, 1990).

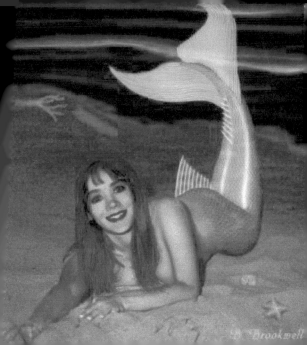

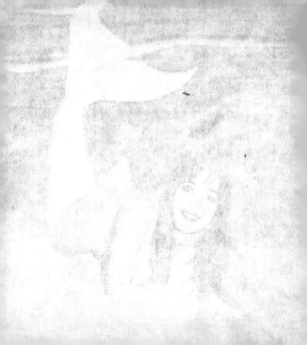

175) Go through your home and office, room by room, and eliminate sources of pollution. Even small changes can improve your health and home.

176) For home safety, stop using toxic products and supplies; begin using safer, alternative products. As consumer demands increase, more companies are offering safer products, such as: cleaning supplies, personal care products, packaged goods and foods, water and air filters, computers, faxes, carpets, padding, and furniture. Test your home for lead, radon, and other hazards. Use inexpensive lead test kits, such as: Leadcheck Swabs, c/o HybriVet Systems, Inc., P.O. Box 1210, Framingham, MA 01701. Call: 1-800-262-LEAD; or The Frandon Lead Alert Kit, c/o Frandon Enterprises, 511 North 48th Street, Seattle, WA 98103. Call: 1-800-359-9000.

177) Buy an effective water filter for your home, especially for your drinking water (such as MultiPure®). Filters can improve taste and make water clear. Depending on the brand, they can remove odors, chlorine, asbestos, microscopic organisms, lead, and other chemicals. Water filters, which remove chlorine, are available for your shower (such as Rainshow'r®). These filters can help to reduce the drying effects of impure water on skin and hair.

178) Improve indoor air quality. Buy and use a high-efficiency air filter to help eliminate dust, spores, bacteria, smoke, and other airborne contaminants. Allow fresh air and sunlight into your home. Open windows to create cross-ventilation. Install a high-quality filter for your heating system; change it regularly or get one that washes clean.

179) Use a low-allergy vacuum cleaner, or one with a water-trap (such as a Rainbow®). Some studies show that these vacuums can effectively trap dirt, dust, and other particles that can cause allergies and illness.

180) Clean and dust regularly. Wear a dust mask. Arrange for help with housework when necessary. Consider bartering with a friend if you cannot afford to hire help. Or explore home-help options with your doctor or a social worker.

181) Use nontoxic, alternative cleaning products. For a general purpose cleaner, use 3 tablespoons baking soda mixed into 1 quart of warm water. For heavy duty cleaning, use Borax in hot water. Clean windows and glass with white vinegar and water, or rubbing alcohol and water. Clean the bathtub and tiles with water and baking soda. Use lemon juice and salt, or white vinegar and salt, to remove mildew. Note: Do not mix cleaning products together; they may become highly toxic.

182)   If you have allergies or are sensitive to chemicals, buy fragrance-free and hypoallergenic products. Many companies offer perfume-free soaps, cleaning products, laundry detergents, deodorants, shampoos, conditioners, and skin care products.

183)   A new home or apartment should be built with non-fuming plywood and particle board that emit less formaldehyde. Use solid wood instead of plywood, plastic, or particle board whenever possible. Avoid the use of tung oil and other irritants. Avoid carpets and carpet padding which contain formaldehyde. Tile or wood floors with area rugs made from natural fibers are safer. An excellent booklet is: *Building Naturally:A Guide to Professionals* by David Kibbey and the Natural Building Network, P.O. Box 1110, Sebastopol, CA 95473.

Reduce Tree- & Plant-Related Allergies

Many people suffer from plant-related allergies. Consequences to health, medical costs, and the economy are tremendous. There has been an increase in new allergy victims; while others with lifelong symptoms have been feeling worse. This is probably related to increasing pollen levels. Greater exposure to allergens often results in increased illness. During the height of pollen season, from late February to June, there can be thousands of pollen grains in every cubic meter of air. You can breathe in hundreds of pollens with each breath. By selecting plants that are least likely to cause allergies, you can enhance your health. Start a community-wide effort to control pollen pollution to help safeguard public health, while reducing health care costs and pain and suffering from allergies.

184) Begin to identify and avoid hazardous, allergy-producing trees, shrubs, plants, weeds, or grasses that may affect you. Avoid trees such as: acacia, alder, ash, birch, cottonwood, elm, oak, olive, pecan, poplar, walnut, and willow. Avoid shrubs such as: elderberry, juniper, and privet. Some allergy-producing weeds are: English plantain, lamb's quarters, pickleweed, pigweed, ragweed, Russian thistle, sheep sorrel, and spiny cockle bur. Grasses to avoid include: annual blue, Bermuda, Kentucky blue, oat, rye, and Timothy.

185) Use potentially "sneezeless" trees, shrubs, ground cover, grass lawn, and ornamental flowers whenever possible. Such trees include: Chinese tallow, tulip tree, silk, silk oak, strawberry, catalpa, pine, pear, podocarpus, dogwood, fir, palm, redwood, fig, jacaranda, plum, crape mytle, coral, orchid, red bud, maidenhair (Gingko), mayten, magnolia, and chorisia. "Sneezeless" shrubs include: nandina, oleander, yucca, manzanita, pyracantha, viburnum, hibiscus, boxwood, and verbena. Ground covers include: cinquefoil, tradescantia, and sedum. Grass lawns include: dichondra, bunch grasses (rye, blue, fescue, etc.), Irish moss, Hippocrepis comosa, and Mazus reptans. Use "sneezeless" ornamental flowers such as: poppy, azalea, camelia, bouganvillea, solanum, cymbidium, begonia, pansy, bulbs (tulip, ranunculus, iris, daffodil, etc.), and peony. Replacing existing plants may be impractical. However, you may plant future gardens using non-allergy trees, plants, shrubs, and flowers. ("Sneezeless Landscaping" pamphlet by the American Lung Association of California and written by Dianna Ricky.)

Chapter 5. Promoting Psychological Health

"Awareness directs thought. Thought directs life-energy, and life-energy follows thought. Where there is pain, from mild to acute, the flow of life-energy is obstructed. Where awareness is focused, the power of life-energy is concentrated."
— *Basic Principles of Actualism*, © 1985 by Russell Paul Schofield, Carol Ann Schofield, and The School of Actualism)

Maintain A Healthy & Optimistic Attitude

Thinking of and feeling love or energy can uplift us in mind and body. Many studies verify that meditation, mindfulness, prayer, and humor can boost the immune system and promote health and a positive attitude. We are what we think. Knowing the power of thought, you can choose positive and loving thoughts about yourself and others. You can learn to let go of negative thoughts which cause *dis*-ease, and begin to think, feel, and act in healthier ways.

Being more conscious of your thoughts, emotions, and actions has many health benefits. Learn what makes you feel good and what makes you uncomfortable. Increase your awareness, keep your focus in the present moment, and pay closer attention to your thoughts, feelings, and body. Choose to maintain a positive perspective, even while going through challenges. Pace yourself and you can balance your energy levels with your activities. Keeping an optimistic outlook and setting healthy limits are fundamental healing principles.

Pessimism, worry, anger, and fear cause stress and "dis-ease," undermining your health and happiness. Worry does not help to resolve anything. It only creates a negative impact on your sense of security, self-esteem, and well-being. Numerous studies show that stress and worry cause a multitude of degenerative problems. Your perspective on life, whether positive or negative, has a great impact on your health. Optimism tends to support your body's ability to heal itself. Developing inner strength and being hopeful can be energizing and empowering.

> Optimism is "an inclination to anticipate the best possible outcome."
> *Webster's Unabridged Dictionary of American English* Third College Ed., 1988

In their book, *Healthy Pleasures* (Addison-Wesley Publishing, 1989), Robert Ornstein, Ph.D. and David Sobel, M.D. write, "Being happy should be easy—we have our pick of sweet smells, sunlight, massages, natural views, and uplifting music. However...we might still find a good mood elusive." The human mind filters, screens, censors, and passes judgment on our overall happiness. The surge from good experiences to good feelings is often blocked by negative thinking. The authors believe that, "An optimist expects good things to happen... this feeling crowds out negativity and seems to improve health. An optimistic frame of mind reshapes the stories we tell ourselves about our past, present, and future. Optimism involves memory. We selectively remember positive events at the expense of negative ones. It involves our current situation: we actively highlight the more promising aspects of the present. It involves the future: looking to a promising tomorrow with an eye toward what can be done instead of what can't happen. People who are positive feel hopeful, not helpless, concerning their future. An optimist feels challenged by the future and its difficulties, believing that he or she can control the environment. An optimist believes that the world is coherent and that individual actions can make a significant difference." Passionately engaged in life, optimists believe in their abilities, they have healthy self-esteem, feel as if they matter, and they may live longer, healthier lives.

Abraham Lincoln said, "A man is as happy as his mind allows him to be." So how can we change our minds to allow ourselves to feel happier? According to Drs. Ornstein and Sobel, "The mind can enhance enjoyment or squelch it. We can influence our wheeling, dealing, changing, churning mind. We need to invest in our mental life in the same way we invest our money or our time. Our minds can shift to allow us greater health and happiness if we learn sound mental investing." Pessimists find that their experiences and life achievements contribute little to their happiness and health. Optimists enjoy life's pleasures.

Focus On What You *Can* Do!

186)   Chronic illness can cause you to experience many losses, such as the loss of energy, health, fitness, career, income, or relationships. When you do not feel well, or when you feel fear or pain, you may tend to focus on problems. Actively seek good medical care, effective emotional and psychological support, and resources to heal and empower you.

187)   See possibilities instead of obstacles. Keep your focus on what you *can* do. Grieve your losses; then let go of what you can no longer do. This shift in focus can help you feel more optimistic about your health.

188)   Face and accept your condition in order to deal with it. Allow yourself to experience your feelings.

189)   Peter McWilliams and John-Roger, authors of *You Can't Afford The Luxury of a Negative Thought*, describe the power of thoughts and their impact on health. Their book is for "people with life-threatening illnesses and for anyone afflicted with one of the primary diseases of our time: negative thinking!"

190)   Make a list and appreciate what is going *right* with your body/health.

191)   If you find yourself stuck in negative thinking, tell yourself, "Stop!" And then substitute positive thoughts about yourself or your life.

192)   Realize that you can learn to train your mind to think positively and to help you to feel better. Cognitive therapists have had much success in treating a variety of psychological problems, including depression, by helping patients reprogram their thoughts.

193)   Changing your outlook can help you to feel better emotionally, psychologically, and physically. Try this exercise. Sit in a comfortable chair and take a few deep breaths. When you feel relaxed, begin to allow positive images about your health to come into your mind. You may be pleasantly surprised at some of these images. If fear or negative thoughts come up, just look at them and let it go. Know that you are in control of your thoughts.

194)   Make a list of things that you would enjoy doing, alone or with others. List places you want to go, people you want to see, books you want to read, restaurants you want to try, or meals you want to prepare. Include whatever things you can do to promote your healing. Then begin to do one thing at a time to create a happier and healthier life. After trying each thing, check it off and write your comments as well.

Psychological Support

195)   Getting the right psychological support is essential when dealing with long-term illness. Don't be shy about telling people what you need and asking for help. When you feel better, you can reciprocate.

196)   Get professional help to deal with all of the emotions associated with chronic illness—such as anger, depression, and fear. Find a caring, supportive, open-minded, and intelligent psychotherapist who can understand your particular challenges and needs regarding your illness. Find someone who is trustworthy—someone with whom you can openly discuss your feelings. Have your therapist help you to heal the complex emotional issues related to your illness. If your therapist does not know about your particular illness, you can bring her or him medical articles, books, or video tapes. (Note: You may need to talk to several therapists until you find one with whom you are most comfortable. Or get a referral from a friend or your doctor.)

197)   Positive support groups, close friends, and "telephone buddies" can make your health problems seem more manageable. Having an ongoing support team, whether in person or on the phone, can create a strong foundation for rebuilding health and for staying hopeful.

198)   Do whatever nurtures you and makes you feel good, whether that means taking a warm bath or taking yourself out to a special dinner.

199)   For health reasons, it is important to talk to yourself in loving, gentle, and nurturing ways. Tell yourself positive statements or write "affirmations" to reprogram your mind to work for you, instead of against you. You can change your mental programming by blocking out criticism from others and from yourself. Learn to release criticism from your mind and body. Criticism serves no useful purpose. Negative thinking causes the subconscious to produces negative results. Negative talk inside your head can defeat you, both mentally and physically. (See "Recommended Reading" list. Books by Dr. Shad Helmstetter and Matthew McKay, Ph.D. are excellent resources.)

200)   Develop an awareness of your critical inner voice. Learn to counterbalance it with a strong healthy voice. Write any criticisms and then write positive statements next to those criticisms. This process can take time and effort but it is well worth the effort. Building a healthy voice is similar to building and toning your muscles, strength, and energy. With practice and dedication, you can trim the fat and get your muscles fit and functioning at peak levels. In a similar manner, you can develop a powerful and positive mental fitness.

Dealing With Depression

Living with a chronic illness can make anyone's life complicated. To make matters worse, well-meaning but confused family members, friends, or even doctors may view your symptoms, fatigue, or illness as "just depression" or "all in your head," (especially when you may be bedridden or when depression is present along with physical symptoms). This type of thinking and lack of understanding or support can undermine your well-being and recovery. It can affect your sense of reality and your self-esteem by causing even you to question the validity of your experience and health problems. While you want people to believe you and to understand, it can be a waste of your precious time and energy trying to convince others that your illness is, in fact, a very real, physical condition—not just a figment of your imagination. Our society tends to want to dismiss certain illnesses; but, unfortunately, this attitude does not make those illnesses go away.

It is natural for anyone faced with a chronic illness to feel depressed at times. People with chronic fatigue tend to maintain their interests, although their energy level may be too low to do all that they want. People with clinical depression tend to lose all interest in activities, as well as have low energy.

201)   Join a support group that makes you feel hopeful, provides you with help and information, and that gives you a sense of community.

202)   To cope with depression, find a compassionate therapist who specializes in the treatment of depression and one who understands your illness or who is willing to learn about it.

203)   Seek professional help if you are feeling severely depressed, helpless, and hopeless. There are a number of effective treatments available today. Seeking help is a sign of strength, not weakness.

204)   Have a long talk with a caring and nurturing friend or relative.

205)   Read *When Feeling Bad Is Good* (Bantam Books, 1994) by Ellen McGrath, Ph.D., a nationally recognized expert on depression. This innovative self-help program teaches women how to convert "healthy" depression into new sources of growth and power.

206)   Read *How To Heal Depression* by Harold H. Bloomfield, M.D. and Peter McWilliams (Los Angeles, CA, Prelude Press, 1994; To order call: 1-800 -LIFE-101). More than 80% of people with depression can be successfully treated with medication and short-term therapy. This simple, direct, compassionate book includes information on: understanding depression; healing the brain and the mind; finding a doctor; getting support; and healing interpersonal relationships.

207)   *The Depression Workbook: A Guide For Living With Depression And Manic Depression* by Mary Ellen Copeland, M.S. with Matthew McKay, Ph.D. (Oakland, CA: New Harbinger Publications, 1992), offers step-by-step, self-help guidance for taking responsibility for your own wellness; using charts to track and control your moods; finding appropriate mental health professionals; building a support system; increasing your confidence and self-esteem; using relaxation, diet, exercise, and full-spectrum light to stabilize your moods; and avoiding conditions that exacerbate mood swings. By reading about others' experiences and learning about current therapeutic strategies, *The Depression Workbook* will give you insight, energy, and hope.

208)   *The Feeling Good Handbook* by David D. Burns, M.D. (N.Y.: Penguin, 1990) offers powerful new techniques and provides step-by-step exercises that help you to cope with the full range of every day problems. Learn ways to free yourself from fears, phobias, and panic attacks; overcome self-defeating attitudes; discover the five secrets of intimate communication; put an end to marital conflict; conquer procrastination; and unleash your potential for success. His book, *Feeling Good: The New Mood Therapy* (William Morrow & Co., 1980), provides a ground-breaking, drug-free treatment for depression.

Empowering & Coping Statements

Write or say aloud any of these "coping" statements (action-oriented statements), which can help you to take charge of your life. Or make up your own empowering statements that are more suitable for your particular needs.

209)   I can take an active role in my own healing and recovery program.
210)   I can find the right doctor to help me achieve my healing goals.
211)   I can choose to eat only nutritious foods that promote healing.
212)   I can eliminate things that cause me to feel bad or make me backslide.
213)   I can decide what is best for my health and then follow that plan.
214)   I can learn skills to take better care of myself, physically and mentally.
215)   I can find new ways to feel more energetic and have more vitality.
216)   I can handle all of the challenges associated with having an illness.
217)   I can take appropriate steps toward improving the quality of my life.
218)   I can develop and maintain an optimistic perspective on my life.
219)   I can have a healthy sense of humor and allow myself to laugh often.
220)   I can see new possibilities, instead of limitations or obstacles.
221)   I can make my life more meaningful by making the most of each day.
222)   I can improve the quality of my relationships with family and friends.
223)   I can learn to assert myself in healthy ways to get my needs met.
224)   I can return kindness for the love and support that I receive.

Affirmations

Write or say "affirmations" (positive statements) about things that you want to work on or improve in your life. Or make up your own. A minister and teacher I know defines affirmations as: "Lies you tell yourself until they become true."

225) I am healing in all ways—in mind, body, emotions, and spirit.
226) I begin to experience more joy and purpose in my life.
227) I am building self-esteem and a strong, nurturing inner voice.
228) I am following what feels right and true for me and my values.
229) I am honest with myself and I express my true feelings to others.
230) I am able to face any challenge directly to solve my problems.
231) I am experiencing more inner peace, harmony, and strength.
232) I am resting and building a reserve of energy for healing.
233) I am able to give and receive love, openly and unconditionally.
234) I am treating myself with respect. I think positively about myself.
235) I approve of myself. I can give up seeking approval from others.
236) I welcome prosperity, creativity, and abundance into my life.
237) I nurture my health, happiness, success, and spiritual growth.
238) I am willing to view my life from a new and positive perspective.
239) I am making progress in all areas of my life, one step at a time.
240) My relationships are becoming more open, loving and nurturing.

Establish Healthy Boundaries

241)   Be aware of what feels positive and healthy to you. Be clear about what is right for you and what fits in with your value system. Also be aware of what feels bad to you or what does *not* fit in with your values.

242)   Learn when to say yes and when to say no. Say yes to things that are right for you. Say no to things that are not right for you. Whether you say yes or no, do not let guilt, fear, or pressure change your answer.

243)   Manuel J. Smith, Ph.D., author of *When I Say No I Feel Guilty: How To Cope—Using The Skills Of Systematic Assertive Therapy* (Bantam Books, 1981), writes about your "bill of assertive rights." He believes that, "You have the right to judge your own behavior, thoughts, and emotions, and to take the responsibility for their initiation and consequences upon yourself. You have the right to offer no reasons or excuses for justifying your behavior. You have the right to judge if you are responsible for finding solutions to other people's problems. You have the right to change your mind. You have the right to be independent of the goodwill of others before coping with them.... You have the right to say no, without feeling guilty."

244) Say yes to the things that you enjoy doing. Say yes to the things that give you energy, make you feel happy, and make you feel good.

245) Say no to invitations to go places if you do not have the energy or if you are not feeling well. You can make plans for another day.

246) Detach from other peoples' negative emotions, depression, or anxiety.

247) If you are in an abusive, destructive relationship, seek professional help immediately and get out of the relationship as soon as possible.

Pace Yourself

248) Plan ahead. Set up an appropriate schedule that works well for you, taking into account any limitations because of illness or low energy.

249) Take frequent breaks throughout the day—whether or not you think that you need them (you probably do).

250) Take several deep breaths and relax when you feel nervous or tense.

251) Pay attention to how you are feeling and take care of your needs.

Build Healthy Self-Esteem

252) Matthew McKay, Ph.D. and Patrick Fanning, co-authors of *Self-Esteem: A Proven Program of Cognitive Techniques for Assessing, Improving, and Maintaining Your Self-Esteem* (Oakland, California: New Harbinger Publications), provide a step-by-step program for quieting our self-critical voices. They teach readers to have compassion for themselves and for others, using hypnosis and visualization for self-acceptance. They suggest that we ask for what we want. And they teach parents how to raise children with high self-esteem.

253) Develop and maintain a positive perspective on your life. See your life filled with new and exciting opportunities for growth. Visualize yourself overcoming obstacles and achieving your goals. Pay attention to how you view yourself. Do things that enhance your self-esteem.

254) Feel good about yourself and other people will respond positively to your healthy sense of self-worth. Be a good role model for them. Let go of self-doubt, criticism, negative thinking, guilt, or skepticism. Release any of your limitations that are fear-based. Focus on your positive qualities and talents. Do not let negative self-images chip away at your health, happiness, or quality of life. Appreciate yourself.

255)   Read Nathaniel Brandon's books on self-esteem.

256)   Nurture your inner child—who deserves your love and support. Build your confidence. And believe that you are worthy and deserving.

257)   Set priorities for your needs and begin to get your needs met. Put your health requirements first. Don't spread yourself too thin. Limit things that drain your energy or make you feel bad.

258)   List your accomplishments, whether small or large. Give yourself credit for any steps taken toward your goals. Keep your list updated. Read it often and feel good about yourself. Reward yourself.

259)   Tell yourself that you now have healthy self-confidence and then allow this belief to become a self-fulfilling prophecy.

260)   Begin to approve of yourself. Self-approval builds self-esteem, inner strength, and happiness. Let go of trying to live up to the expectations of others, which is a stressful burden. Forget about seeking approval from other people, which makes you focus outside of yourself.

261)   Recreate your life according to your own specific dreams and desires.

Dream Therapy

"There are many common themes in our dreams," according to Dr. Alan Siegel, psychotherapist and author of *Dreams That Can Change Your Life* (Berkley Books, 1990). People often dream of car crashes, which may represent feelings of crashing emotionally. We often dream about the past or the future. If you dream that you have an illness that has not materialized yet, your subconscious may be warning you to take better care of yourself. Dr. Siegel writes, "Many people dream they are being chased by wild animals, which can represent fear, depression, or anxiety. Troubling dreams often disrupt our sleep. Repressed memories come through dreams. What you dream doesn't necessarily mean that it happened or that it will happen, although you can explore the ideas."

"Dreams can help us navigate a smoother course through the emotional turbulence of life's turning points," says Dr. Siegel. Dreams can change our lives by allowing us to identify and reclaim powerful hidden feelings that undermine our ability to move forward. They show us what stage we have reached in adapting to a major turning point and provide us with an accurate gauge of the inner changes that occur. They warn us about emotional conflicts and self-defeating behaviors that block our ability to cope with change. They help us identify and resolve past wounds and anxieties that have resurfaced to plague us in the present. Dreams can point to solutions to an emotional impasse. They can confirm our success at resolving the challenges of a turning point. They help us to see the importance of reaching out to others for crucial emotional support at times of change. They allow us to perceive solutions to conflicts in our close relationships. They get us in touch with new sources of creativity in our work and inspire new directions and projects. Dreams can restore a sense of meaning and instill hope—helping us make it through tough times.

262) Keep a journal to help analyze your dreams. Title each dream. Use a dream analysis book for guidance. Talk into a tape recorder or write down your dreams as soon as you wake up. This will help you to remember more of the details. Or tell your lover or friend about them.

263) Look for common themes in your dreams. Then link your dreams to your feelings, health, and life. Look for any images or symbolism. What do your dreams represent or reveal to you? Look for recurring dreams. Dr. Siegel says that, "Recurring dreams are dramatic messages from your subconscious mind."

264) Program your dreams by giving yourself mental suggestions before you fall asleep. Your dreams will tell you about yourself. Ask yourself questions about what you need to know. Ask: What benefits will this dream have for me? What answer will it provide? Answers often come through in symbols. Discover what these symbols mean to you. You may need to change thoughts into symbols to understand your dreams. (Artists and scientists use symbols to study and resolve problems.)

265) Program yourself to remember your dreams more clearly. Before sleeping, ask that your dreams help to heal your pain or past trauma. Ask that your dreams reveal ways in which you can promote healing.

266) Make or buy an "Indian Dream Catcher." Native Americans believed that dreams, both good and bad, descended from the night sky. Bad dreams were captured in a web and then held there until the morning sun rays could evaporate them. Good dreams could slip through the web onto the dreamer.

Classes & Workshops For Self-Enrichment

267) Begin a personal self-enrichment program. Get involved with health education and preventive medicine. Your doctor may be able to refer you to a health education class. Attending a class is a good way to meet supportive people while enhancing your health and your life.

268)   At times you may experience a lack of time, energy, help, or money. Yet with a little effort, you can gather an abundance of information and resources to guide and inform you. You probably have access to a wide range of free or low-cost classes, workshops, and lectures. You may learn from documentaries, self-help and medical books, audio and video tapes, computers, and hotline services. Government agencies may also offer you assistance, referrals, and information.

269)   Take a class or workshop. Or attend a lecture at a local hospital, community center, college, or university. You may benefit from taking classes on: stress reduction, healthy cooking, nutrition, weight control, exercise, meditation, yoga, prenatal care, parenting, heart health, art/music therapy, or other healing programs. Or you may need help to stop abuse or to end an addiction to drugs, alcohol, or smoking.

270)   Take a writing class. Begin working on the book that you have always wanted to write. Or try a screenwriting class. Have students read your work aloud so you can hear how the dialog sounds. Or write and act out a play with a friend. Writing and acting can be healing.

Chapter 6. Promoting Emotional Health

Being as optimistic as possible is good for your health; however, it is important for mental and physical well-being to acknowledge your true thoughts and feelings. So do not deny or ignore any pain or discomfort that you may be experiencing. Instead, deal with your emotions directly. If you feel sad or depressed, it is better to face those feelings and work through them. You may want professional counseling for help with this process. Sometimes, you may want to "go around" certain feelings, but that does not make them go away. For example, trying to cope with depression by drinking alcohol or taking illegal drugs often makes the depression worse and sets up a vicious cycle.

In his book, *What You Feel, You Can Heal* (Heart Publishing, 1994), John Gray, Ph.D. writes, "The ability to feel emotion is a gift we all share as human beings. Often you may not like what you are feeling. Every emotion has a purpose and that emotion will remain with you until that purpose is realized and understood. Your feelings are like messengers from your subconscious to your conscious mind. Until you receive the message, the messenger will stand patiently at your door. What are the messages your feelings bring to you? Anger arises to tell you that what is happening to you is undesirable. Hurt or sadness arises to tell you that you have lost or are missing something you want or need. Fear arises to warn you of the possibility of failure, loss, or pain. Guilt arises to remind you that... you are responsible for causing an undesirable circumstance."

"The way to understand your emotions and what they are telling you about your life is to express them," says Dr. Gray. "You cannot understand what remains unexpressed. Through expressing the complete truth about all of your feelings, you can eventually realize the loving intention underneath all of your negative emotions.... Your mind and body are intimately connected. Each is there to serve the other. If you choose to repress an uncomfortable emotion, your body may try to 'help' resolve the tension you've created by releasing that tension for you through various physical symptoms." (Popular ways of avoiding feelings include overeating; overshopping; and excessive drinking, smoking, and gambling.)

Dr. Gray lists several physical symptoms which are often related to the emotional dis-ease people may be feeling, such as: Muscular tension: "He's a pain in the neck." Headache: "I don't want to think about it anymore." Viruses and colds: "I've decided to act cold to her." Arthritis: "I was scared stiff" or "I guess I'm just set in my ways." High Blood Pressure: "He really blew his top" or "I'm under so much pressure." Respiratory: "I feel like this job is suffocating me." Constipation: "I can't seem to let go of the past." Heart Disease: "She broke my heart." And, Fever: "He has a hot temper." Are you experiencing any physical symptoms which may be related to your emotions?

271) An open mind and an open heart help to nurture your emotional health. Seeing the "bigger picture" of your life provides a healthier perspective. Believe in and experience your life's miracles. For example, directly experience your life energy by feeling your pulse, listening to your heart beat, and feeling more passion or joy. Focus on what's right with your body. Your body will respond to love, laughter, nurturing, proper nutrition, fresh air, clean water, and sunlight—just as plants and trees flourish when they receive water, proper soil, air, and light. You can add more healing elements to your environment. Choose to invite a fun-loving friend over for a healthy meal or spend more time with your children. Discovering and doing what makes you feel good are steps toward creating more happiness.

Emotional Support

272) Ongoing support of a group (such as a 12-Step program or therapy group) can help you take a closer, more honest look at yourself and your life. Positive support makes getting to know yourself and looking within less scary. With nurturing support, you can explore and deal with emotionally-charged issues, thoughts, or experiences. By opening up and sharing your feelings and personal problems in a safe and caring environment, you can work though any anger, emptiness, fear, or pain. You may find it helpful to write a journal about what you learn. Ongoing, positive support can empower you to make life-enhancing changes. It can put you on a new track so that you can create a healthy new train of thoughts, feelings, and actions.

273)   Read a self-help book that you find meaningful and enjoyable. Discuss what you have read with a friend or a support person. You may want to read the book together and discuss related experiences as you read. Exploring and expressing thoughts and feelings about the material helps you to clarify and personalize it. Allow yourself to feel any feelings that come up as you read. Share insights, feelings, or ideas that are meaningful or uplifting. Write about these experiences.

274)   Sit alone for a while in a quiet, comfortable room. Ask yourself what you really need to feel better emotionally. Make a list of your needs. Then, one by one, begin to take care of those needs yourself or get help. Keep your list handy, and check off each need as it is fulfilled.

275)   Develop new compassion for yourself. Have patience. Find ways to release painful emotional layers that may be blocking your feelings and zest for life.

276)   Explore ways of finding help and inspiration to break through any stubborn old emotional blocks, which may be keeping you from feeling emotionally healthy and happy. With the right support, you can learn to let go of fear, feel your feelings, and manage and enjoy your life.

277)   Get professional help to deal with any anger or rage that you may feel regarding any losses or complications associated with your illness. Grieve any losses you may have experienced. Have a good cry (often).

278)   Allow yourself to feel any fear, resentment, or suppressed emotions. Work through any upsetting feelings and cleanse yourself of them. Replace any negative emotions with self-love, respect, and acceptance.

279)   Have a "pity party" with a friend or support group. Allow each person to openly and honestly express his or her feelings or complaints for two minutes, without any interruptions. Then give each person time (another two minutes) to list things for which he or she is grateful.

280)   Practice "smile" therapy, even though you may be alone or not in the mood. Sometimes if you just smile, you will automatically feel better. Surround yourself with positive, happy, and supportive people.

281) Learn from your illness by discovering what brings more harmony into your body, mind, emotions, life, and spirit. Encourage more positive thoughts and feelings. Be kind and loving to yourself. Think loving thoughts about your body. Appreciate how well your body does function. Make a list of your healthy qualities, attitudes, and feelings.

282) Sun Bear (a medicine chief of the Bear Tribe Medicine Society based in Spokane, Washington and author of *Sun Bear: The Path of Power* and *The Medicine Wheel*) helps people let go of their negative feelings. He instructs each person to go out and dig a hole in the earth. Speaking upsetting feelings into that hole, he or she dumps out previously unexpressed rage, grief, dread, or sickness. This process helps people to release negativity and gain a sense of well-being.

283) Examine and express your feelings, and let loved ones express their feelings. Illness can strain communication and honesty can be healing.

Telephone Buddies

284) Call a telephone hotline service or a foundation which provides support and information regarding your illness. Ask if they have a list of support groups or telephone support buddies you may contact.

285) Find a support person—someone you feel comfortable with and possibly someone who is experiencing the same illness. Ask if he or she is interested in developing a mutually-supportive relationship in person or over the telephone. When you feel lonely or isolated from being house-bound, call your phone buddy. Have a heart-to-heart talk.

286) Having a support person and being there for each other over a period of time can make a big difference in both of your lives.

287) If your phone buddy does not live in your community, you may want to call the telephone company and ask if they have special rates. Some companies offer special discounts to low income households or to people with disabilities. Other companies may offer discounts on calls made to one particular person or area. Using the phone can help you feel less isolated but make sure you don't cause stress by accumulating high phone bills.

Positive Support Groups

Participating in a support group that deals directly with your particular illness can be beneficial in many ways. You can learn how others are coping with your illness and the group can offer you referrals to good doctors and resources.

Sharing and exploring personal feelings, grief, and pain in a supportive group can help you to release fears, anxiety, and stress. People are encouraged when they feel that they are not "alone." The right support group can help you to gain insight, strength, and coping skills by learning how others are handling similar problems. Many studies now confirm that support groups help promote healing.

Support Group Tips

288)   Call a local hospital, organization, foundation, or hotline service that provides information about your illness. Ask if they know of a support group in your area. Or ask your doctor, therapist, or friends for a referral to a group that will offer you help, support, and information.

289)   When you find a support group, call the facilitator and schedule an interview. You may want to ask him or her these questions: What is your background/experience? Do you have a degree? What does the group involve? What are the guidelines? What is the focus of the meetings? Is the group free? If there is a charge (and if you are limited on funds) is there a sliding pay scale? How many people are in the group? Is the group open or must members make a commitment to attend the group for a period of time? Ask any other questions that are important for you to know.

290)   Before making a commitment to a group, you may want to attend a few meetings to see how you feel about it. Be sure the group you join has an effective group leader, one who can keep the group on track and focused on healing and supportive communication. A group should feel "safe." The facilitator should establish trust and confidentiality.

Facilitating Your Own Support Group

You may want to start a group for people who are dealing with similar health problems. You may want to get together with a group of positive people once a week to share your thoughts, feelings, and support. Or you may decide to form a group for art or humor therapy, goal-setting, brainstorming or problem-solving. Being a group facilitator can be a challenging and rewarding experience. It is an excellent way for you to help others, while helping yourself.

291)   Begin taking steps to create a support group for healing. It may be easier to create a group with a friend or a support person. Or find an organization or health care professional to help you get started. Write a wish list for your group. What do you need? What will it be like? How will it be structured? What is the group's focus? What do you want your group to accomplish? Where will it be held? And, when?

292)   Make a list of positive and supportive people who would be an asset to your group. List people who may be interested in joining because they want support dealing with a similar illness. Begin contacting people. Ask if they would like to join a support group with a focus on healing. If they do, ask them what day and time they could meet. Choose a time that works for the majority of the people. A two-hour meeting, once a week, is usually appropriate. Choose someone to be your assistant. Call local churches, libraries, community centers, or schools to find a free or low-cost meeting room that is conveniently located. Choose a room that is accessible to those who are disabled or in wheelchairs. Choose a comfortable, light, and cheerful room; ideally, one with temperature controls.

293)   Prepare for your group by writing the group's focus and purpose. The focus might include these concepts: 1) Healing/empowering ourselves; 2) Support through care and understanding; or 3) Building our self-esteem. The group's purpose, or mission statement, might include: 1) To share information, resources, and tips for coping with illness; 2) To empower each other; 3) To problem-solve; 4) To help us build strength; or 5) To establish a phone list for keeping in touch and creating a buddy system. Note: You may revise the focus or purpose as the group evolves.

294)   Write a list of goals and guidelines for your group. Here are some important examples: Confidentiality should be respected. (Members may discuss their own or others' ideas and/or experiences outside the group as long as no names or clues to the identity of people are revealed.) A phone list of members can be made available for people who wish to contact each other outside of the group for additional support or information. Individuals should not wear perfume or fragrances to the group because members may have chemical sensitivities. No smoking is allowed in the group meeting. During "sharing" or "check-ins" everyone is allowed to speak without being interrupted for a certain amount of time. Begin with 2 minutes each.

295)   To begin a group meeting, welcome members, introduce yourself, and talk briefly about your background. Explain the focus, purpose, structure, and format of the group. You may provide a written outline for clarity. Offer some words of encouragement to set the tone of the meeting—read a quote or a poem, share some inspiring news, or sing a song. Explain some basic guidelines. For example, "This is an opportunity to share our needs and insights with each other. Together, we can create a safe place to be heard and understood. We can help inspire each other in positive, healing ways and share what bothers us and get support. Yet we will not spend all of our time focused on negative, depressing issues because we may feel overwhelmed and discouraged. So let's keep a healthy balance of expressing our needs and discussing possible options." Pass around a telephone list for anyone who wants to receive calls. Take a few moments to make any relevant announcements or share health care tips or information.

296) During the discussion part of the group, set a time limit for individual sharing. Divide the time up equally. It is usually best not to let one person dominate the group, especially if he or she is very upset. This can upset the group and throw everyone off track. If anyone is feeling anxious or depressed, you can talk to him or her after the meeting.

297) After individual sharing, you may choose a topic and have a general discussion. Talk about the next meeting and encourage members to mark the date on their calendars. To close the group, read something inspirational, sing an uplifting song (such as "Amazing Grace"), or say a prayer or an affirmation together. Thank members for coming.

298) Learn to become an effective group leader. They are well organized. They have good communication skills and good "people" skills. They are good listeners and they motivate people. Effective group leaders help to solve problems, establish trust and cooperation, and delegate responsibilities. They empower the group by maintaining a sense of fairness and an awareness of individual needs. They get input from the group and they help to make clear decisions. They keep the group on track by setting healthy limits and keeping the group upbeat.

299) Limit the number of members for your group (6 to 8 people is ideal). Members should agree to: being committed to the group, attending meetings regularly, and calling the facilitator when they can't attend.

300) To empower others and yourself in a group, "speak from the heart." Use encouraging statements such as: What a great idea! Glad to hear it! You can do it! Good for you. That's really wonderful! How exciting!

Dealing With Anger

Chronic illness can make you feel frustrated and angry. You can become very sick and tired of feeling sick and tired. But frequent anger can take a heavy toll on your mental, physical, and emotional well-being as it causes stress and anxiety. Studies show that anger can even become life-threatening. Therefore, it is essential for your health to learn effective and appropriate ways to deal with anger. One way is to practice "coping skills." Or repeat coping statements to yourself, such as: "I am coping with pain and stress in the best ways I can."

301)   Work with a therapist or follow the exercises recommended in the book, *When Anger Hurts: Quieting The Storm Within*, by M. McKay, P. D. Rogers, and J. McKay (New Harbinger Publications, 1989). The authors write, "Whether you are learning stress reduction or a system to alter your anger-triggering thoughts, this book can only help if you master each step and then apply what you've learned to real events in your life. The work will pay off." The authors believe that coping skills can help you to achieve healthy benefits, including: 1) The ability to control destructive anger venting. Learn to protect and rebuild relationships that may have been damaged by venting anger in the past. 2) Reducing the frequency and intensity of your physiological anger response. Research shows that anger damages your health. The less anger you experience, the longer you may live. 3) A change in beliefs, assumptions, and attitudes that trigger chronic anger. Learn to restructure anger-triggering thoughts and fewer things will upset you. 4) Identifying stresses and needs that lie below your anger. Becoming clear about a problem can move you past anger to decision making. 5) The ability to cope effectively with stress. Instead of exploding when stress exceeds your tolerance threshold, use relaxation tools. 6) Greater effectiveness in meeting your needs. Anger generates resistance and resentment in others. When you are angry, you may get short-term cooperation but in the long run, your needs will be ignored and you will be avoided. Problem solving and clear communication will help you get what you want without anger.

302)   Keep a journal to record your observations about any anger you may experience. Write about how to best deal with anger. A journal helps you explore any patterns of tension in your body.

303)   Make a list of specific things that make you angry. Allow yourself to feel your feelings. Then work to resolve the situations, one by one, with a friend, a therapist, or a support group.

304)   Assert yourself in appropriate ways and learn to establish healthy personal boundaries. Then you can experience less anger in your life.

305)   Replace anger and frustration with forgiveness and love. Release any anger in your relationships by clearly expressing your needs and by working together to resolve problems.

306)   To release anger, hit a punching bag or a big soft pillow. Yell "Take that!" or "Anger, go away!" or say any phrase that makes you feel a deep sense of release. Cry when you need to. Or laugh. Laughter is a great antidote to anger. You can't frown and laugh at the same time.

307) Play an easy game of tennis or racquetball, even if you can only play for a short time. If you can't find a partner, hit the ball against a wall. Take this opportunity to release your anger as you hit the ball.

308) Keep a journal. Jot down anything that angers you throughout the day. Once a week talk to a therapist or a friend about things in your journal that bother you the most. Get support to resolve your conflicts.

309) Pay close attention to how you feel around people. Some people may make you feel happy or energized; others may tend to make you feel angry or upset. Tell people how you feel, without verbally attacking them. Instead of saying "you made me feel bad" or "you hurt me," you can say, "I feel (hurt, sad, upset, etc.) when you say (_____)." Then ask if you can talk to each other in more nurturing ways. Don't tolerate verbal abuse (Read *The Verbally Abusive Relationship* by P. Evans.)

310) Meditate in a quiet room in your home or in a natural setting. Center yourself. Close your eyes or focus your attention on an object. Relax. Breathe slowly and deeply for several minutes. Experience your inner thoughts, feelings, and the environment. Are you feeling peaceful yet? Keep meditating and you may begin to feel a release of anger or stress. Completely let go and feel a sense of joy and inner peace.

Dealing With Isolation

Studies show that human interaction is good for your health. Social involvement has been found to decrease health risks, while contributing to health benefits.

311)   In her book, *Alone, Alive & Well: How To Fight Loneliness and Win* (Rodale Press, 1985; ISBN 0-87857-574-X), Barbara Powell, Ph.D. suggests ways to enjoy being alone without feeling lonely. Statistics show that loneliness can lead to an increased risk of physical and psychological illness, including severe depression. But statistics may not point out how thousands of people are living alone, alive, and well. Many people who live alone enjoy healthy, active, productive lives. You can learn to appreciate your personal space and begin to enjoy time alone. Dr. Powell says, "Aloneness is not depressing; solitude can be enriching. [People] who live alone but are healthy and happy accept and enjoy their solitude. And they are connected to others by individual relationships and by active group involvements."

312)   Change your attitude about aloneness. Dr. Powell believes that there are three general aspects to staying well and happy while living alone. 1) The need to change negative loneliness into positive solitude. Single people who live happily are not afraid to spend time alone; they cherish their time for private activities. They take time to paint, write, sew, read, or garden without the need to share that precious space. 2) The need to establish a sense of belonging through group membership. Too much solitude can become too much of a good thing. Living alone does not mean being alone all the time. We thrive on a sense of community, on knowing that we belong to a family, a church, or some other close group that will support us in hard times. 3) There is the need to create a strong one-to-one relationship with at least one other person. For most people, the most intense and desirable relationship is one with a spouse or a lover. Dr. Powell says, "Generally, the three aspects of overcoming loneliness move in a natural progression. You must feel comfortable being alone by developing more positive attitudes about yourself and finding some activities you can enjoy by yourself, before you begin to establish a network of casual friends. When you become comfortable in casual relationships, you will be ready to develop greater intimacy with another person."

313) Dr. Robert Weiss of M.I.T., a sociologist who has studied loneliness since the 1960s, believes that both kinds of connection—the group and the intimate—are essential and that one cannot replace the other. He characterizes the absence of a close emotional attachment as "the loneliness of emotional isolation" and the absence of a social network as "social isolation." Viewing loneliness as distinct from depression, he says, "In loneliness there is a drive to rid oneself of one's distress by integrating a new relationship or regaining a lost one; in depression there is instead a surrender to it. The lonely are driven to find others, and if they find the right others, they change and are no longer lonely." Not everyone agrees with this distinction; yet, most researchers believe that being lonely can be both a cause and a consequence of being depressed. One may also be depressed without being lonely.

314)   Get together with a group of people once a month. Hold an informal talent show. Sing, dance, and play musical instruments. Tell jokes. Or share your favorite recipes, poetry, stories, music, art, or games.

315)   Make good use of your time alone. Rest, nurture yourself, meditate, exercise, get to know yourself better, cook a healthy meal, enjoy your hobbies, write letters to loved ones, or take care of your plants.

316)   Try to meet new people and develop friendships at work, school, or church. Build friendships that are mutually respectful and supportive. If your illness has made it difficult for you to work, or if you are often house-bound, there are still many ways you can meet people. Create a sense of "belonging" by joining a support group or finding a support person. Talk to your family members, friends, doctor, or caregivers about ways that you can set up effective support.

317)   Listen to an informative and interesting radio or TV talk show. They can give you a sense of community. Call in and voice your opinion. Even though millions of people may be listening, relax and be yourself.

318)   Invite a few friends over to watch a good film or read a good book. Then share your film or book reviews.

319)   Meet with a friend once a week. Make a wish-list for each person. Work together to make your goals and wishes come true. Give each other little gifts (such as reward stickers) for all accomplishments.

320)   Surround yourself with the things you care about most, such as your favorite books, music, hobbies, photographs, flowers, or animals. Become more involved in hobbies and share them with your friends.

Laughter & Healing

"Laughter eloquently illustrates the mind/body connection." (Benson, 276) You can see connections between laughter, thoughts, postures, and body sensations.

For example, tickling can trigger laughter and so can a funny thought. The late Norman Cousins noted a relationship between the remission of his illness and the laughter he enjoyed while watching humorous videos. He called these healing processes "internal jogging." Many researchers have found that laughter uplifts the spirit and boosts the immune system. Use some of the following tips, or make up your own, to discover what makes you laugh and feel good.

321) Dr. Barrie Greiff, formerly a psychiatrist at the Harvard Business School, believes that a positive approach to life correlates with health and happiness. He suggests advantageous personal habits or his "Five L's of success": Learn, Labor, Love, Laugh, Let go (which allow you to embrace life with involvement, challenge, empowerment, and fun). Approach each day as a chance to Learn (be open to new experiences), Labor (at something that satisfies you and brings meaning to your life), Love (give, recognize, and receive), Laugh (with yourself and others), and Let go (release things that are out of your control). Then the stresses you encounter will seem more manageable. Laughter and a positive attitude will improve how you view a situation and improve your perception of how well you cope. (Benson, 179).

322) Malcolm Kushner, a top "humor consultant" and author of *The Light Touch*, describes ways to use humor to manage your work, health, and life. Humor can be used to help manage conflict and stress, to motivate people, to handle awkward situations, and to improve work and productivity. He provides simple techniques that anyone can use. You don't have to be a comedian and you don't have to be naturally funny. You don't even have to know how to tell a joke. Many techniques can be used without saying a word—such as hanging up a funny sign, poster, or cartoon on your wall. Or create a humor bulletin board, with jokes, cartoons, or photographs. "Humor is a winning strategy," says Kushner. "Humor's ability to change perspective makes it a valuable asset in the battle against stress, an ever-growing problem. By directing comic vision inward, you can change your perceptions of stressful situations and secure a degree of momentary calm."

323) Exchange gag gifts with friends or family members. Create a humor action plan to integrate humor into your life.

324) Read the humor section in national magazines.

325) Rent a few funny and uplifting movies. Invite some fun-loving friends over for a potluck and comedy film festival. Ask everyone to wear a funny costume or a silly hat, wig, mask, or disguise. And ask them to bring enjoyable or silly snacks if they can.

326)   Make some fun party snacks. Here are a few ideas. Prepare pancakes in the shape of cartoon characters or create your friends' initials (by slowly pouring batter onto the frying pan in creative shapes or letters). Bake healthy cookies and use funny cookie cutters. Make a Jello™ mold and try adding fruit cut into silly shapes.

327)   Subscribe to Cable TV and watch the Comedy channel. Listen to some good comedy on the radio. Or go to a comedy club.

328)   Become a "humor consultant" to your family and friends. Learn some funny songs and teach others to sing them. Use a singing machine and record your voices. Or learn great jokes and share them. Teach others to enjoy more humor in their lives.

329)   Go to a used bookstore and buy several joke books, comics, humor magazines, or cassette tapes of your favorite comedians.

330)   Go for a walk or a picnic with a funny friend—one who makes you feel good about yourself and who cheers you up.

331)   Call someone who is ill or feeling depressed and make them laugh and cheer them up.

332) Write a humorous short story or magazine article about a personal experience. Send it to a newspaper or magazine editor.

333) Write and illustrate a humorous children's story. Read it to children and ask for their opinions. Ask them how you can make it funnier.

334) Write your favorite one-liners in a notebook, scrapbook, or joke book. Or make up your own jokes. Include colorful stickers, cartoons, and humorous photos or drawings in your book to liven it up. Keep adding to your collection and share it with others.

335) Fax some of your favorite cartoons or jokes to your friends.

336) Create a "humor happy hour" three times a week.

337) Meet with friends who enjoy good humor. Trade jokes and cartoons.

338) Start a lively support group with the theme: "Laughter & Healing." Have your group create a joke book and use it as your manual.

339) Throw a "surprise" party for yourself. Invite friends over to celebrate your birthday or any other occasion you wish to enjoy with others.

340) Get together with a writing buddy each week. Create a humorous screenplay, an episode for your favorite comedy show, or make up your own situational comedy. Try writing a humor book or a romantic comedy about your life. Or write an article about the lighter side of dealing with illness and share it with others who are ill.

341) Visit people in a nursing home or hospice. Share a joke book or cartoon collection with them.

342) Write about a funny personal experience, or make up a list of jokes, and send them to your favorite talk show host or comedian.

343) Spend more quality time with adults and children who are usually happy and who love to laugh and play.

344) Using bright and colorful chalk, crayons, or finger paints, create funny pictures to hang up on your refrigerator door or on a wall. Do this project with a child or enjoy it with your own "inner child."

345) Go "out on a limb" with your humor. Find ways to make others laugh.

346) Watch your favorite cartoons and draw characters from them.

347)   Create a funny outgoing message on your telephone answering machine. Use music on your message as well.

348)   Create funny greeting cards for your family and friends. Sell them to a hospital gift shop or give them to patients.

349)   Call a close friend who has a good sense of humor. Take turns sharing any funny experiences that you had that day. Or visit friends or family members who are feeling blue and cheer them up.

Pet Therapy

People have enjoyed pets for thousands of years. Recent studies have shown positive and healing results from the relationship between people and companion animals. Pets can inspire us to exercise more and can help us to relax. They can help to build our self-esteem or comfort us when we feel down. Pets help us to open up and communicate with each other. In fact, some people are more comfortable talking to animals than to other people. Pets may help to shorten the recovery time from illness or surgery. They may help to slow the progression of disease, and they may help to reduce the risk of stress-related illnesses, such as heart disease.

Researchers are discovering that watching or petting friendly animals can produce a deep relaxation, similar to meditation, biofeedback, or hypnosis. This response can lower blood pressure. Pet therapy is often used to combat the isolation and loneliness so common in nursing homes. (*Your Emotional Health and Well-Being*. Editors of *Prevention* ® Magazine. Longmeadow Press, 1989.)

Note: Pet therapy does have its limitations and it may not be for everyone. People should select appropriate animals as pets. Be aware that animals may cause allergies, infections, or injuries. For more information on pet therapy, call the Delta Society in the Seattle, Washington area at: (206) 226-7357.

350)   If you feel stressed, ill, alone, isolated, or depressed, consider getting a pet. Spend time with animals and pay attention to how they make you feel. If you do not want the responsibility or expense of caring for a pet, or if you have allergies which prevent you from living with pets, you may enjoy visiting a zoo or doing some volunteer work there.

351)   If you have a cat or a dog, take it for a walk whenever you can.

352)   If you cannot have large pets in your apartment or home, consider getting smaller pets—such as fish, birds, or hamsters. These can be easier to care for, and they can be fun and relaxing to watch.

353)   Virginia Wells, author of *50 All Natural Stress Busters*, writes: "Pets are **fur** hugging. Pets can make you feel happy in a variety of ways. They give you unconditional love, they do not judge you, and they feel nice to the touch. Most pets require a simple diet. They are easily trained to behave by your rules. Pets can inspire you to get out of the house and they love it when you come home. They are good listeners and they do not offer you unwanted advice. They keep you company so you never have to eat or sleep alone. Pets respond to your touch."

354)   If you have a pet, spend more quality time with it. Make a healthy snack for you and your pet. Watch TV or listen to music together.

355)   Take care of a friend's pet for a while, during his or her vacation. This can help you to decide whether or not it is beneficial, enjoyable, or practical for you to own a pet.

356)   Consider getting a pet from an animal shelter. Shelters often need temporary homes for puppies or kittens who need to be socialized. Dogs can be trained to help people with various disabilities.

357)   When you feel sad, lonely, upset, or in need of support, talk to your pet and allow it to comfort you.

Chapter 7. Creative Therapies For Healing

Creativity, joy, and playfulness can enhance your personal growth and self-healing. These activities may help to reduce your stress and anxiety, clarify and express your thoughts and feelings, and uplift your spirits. Drawing, painting, playing music, singing, or dancing are some of the ways you may explore your creative talents. Discover what is rewarding for you, artistically and emotionally.

Art Therapy

Art provides a powerful medium for personal expression and self-discovery. Art therapy is often beneficial for exploring and expressing inner feelings, dreams, visions, and symbols; as well as for exploring issues of intimacy, self-esteem, spirituality, sexuality, grieving, or healing.

"Art is a language that can bypass rational thought and serve as a doorway into deep intuitive knowing," according to Anastasia Horn, M.A., MFCC and Julia Whitney, Ph.D. They state, "Our creations can become powerful catalysts for understanding ourselves and our processes. Art therapy is about giving expression to the inner self in a nonverbal way. It is not about artistic skill or creating visual masterpieces."

"Creative Painting is not just another subject to be learned, it is a living process that happens between us and the painting. Its value lies in the inner movement of events and feelings, not in the result," according to Michell Cassou (founder of an original approach to creative painting used as a tool for self-discovery. She and Stewart Cubley have been teaching in the San Francisco Bay Area for over 17 years). "Emphasis is placed upon the practical experience of creative painting, where people are given support and stimulation to touch deeper in themselves and dissolve creative blocks. The mechanisms and patterns that prevent creative expression are explored in order to discover a natural experience of painting based directly upon feelings."

358)   Talk to your doctor or therapist about attending an art therapy class.

359)   Get a blank drawing paper or a blank canvas. Visualize the new life that you want to create. Then paint your new life with brilliant colors.

360)   Invite a friend over, play some soothing music, and draw or paint. Critique each other's work in positive and supportive terms.

361)   Listen to a guided imagery or visualization tape, and then draw or paint some of the images. Or make up your own creative or therapeutic visualization exercise, and then draw or paint your experience.

362)   Frieda Porat, Ph.D., psychotherapist in the San Francisco Bay Area, created the following therapeutic art exercise. Relax comfortably in a chair and take a few deep breaths. Visualize yourself walking into a long dark tunnel, where you will be perfectly safe. See various doors along the walls of the tunnel. Walk toward the first door on the left and enter the room. Once inside, allow yourself to experience any anger you may feel. What is happening? What or who do you see? Now visualize leaving this room. Walking through the tunnel, find another door on the right and open it. Enter this room and experience any fear. What or whom do you see? Leave this room and walk back to the tunnel. Walk toward a light you see, allowing it to guide you. As you walk out of the tunnel and into warm sunlight, you enter a lush, beautiful garden. You are surrounded by brilliant, colorful flowers and lush exotic plants. Sit on the grass and enjoy the scenery. Begin to come back to your present reality. Slowly open your eyes when you are ready. Draw or paint what you have experienced inside the tunnel and in the garden.

363)   Read *Art As Healing* by Edward Adamson (Boston: Coventure, Ltd., 1990). The author explores these ideas: "The arts have always been associated with spiritual regeneration. The visual arts can be a vital form of self-help, which allows nature's healing powers to restore balance and harmony to the troubled mind. There are many parallels between the dynamics of spontaneous painting and the therapeutic process. Art is a very powerful form of communication, which in turn is a vital part of the therapeutic situation. Painting can be used actively to encourage the person to dream on paper, or to complete an interrupted dream. The act of painting, in itself, is a magical moment. In a therapeutic session, the sensitive doctor can make use of symbolic material in painting, as it is presented. Art gives palpable form to the imagination. The spectator is given the great privilege of being allowed into the secret garden of dreams. Painting gives great satisfaction and pleasure to many people. There seems to be a natural, 'fullness of time' which occurs in both art and healing. Just as a painting cannot be forced, healing must proceed at its own pace. One is obliged to co-operate with this rhythm to avoid any precipitous insult which could abort the process. Art obliges us to communicate with the inner self, and in so doing, to engage in a dialog with both our destructive and creative forces. The destructive powers have precipitated the problem, so that the symptoms of illness we observe are merely the acting out of an unresolved, inward struggle. This knot is more effectively untied by the creative powers of healing art."

Color Therapy

In their book, *Living Color, Master Lin Yun's Guide to Feng Shui and the Art of Color* (Kodansha Int., 1994), Sarah Rossback and Lin Yun offer ways that color can restore and enhance energy, balance, and good fortune in your home and life. Colors are the key to the Chinese art of feng shui ("fung shway"), a system of placement whose simplicity and ecological good sense have struck a cord in the West. Learn to use color application in all areas of your life: home, garden, clothes, food, environment, health, and relationships. The authors teach rules for a balanced, harmonious life based on Tao—the way of all living things. Their research was a treasure hunt, as they explored, examined, and pieced together Chinese philosophy, religion, art, medicine, design, and culture. They believe that color influences our lives and world, defining what exists and what does not exist. It discloses the status of one's health and fortunes. Traditional Chinese doctors are versed in reading the color of one's face or one's chi (energy). Color inspires emotion and influences behavior. Through wise arrangement of color in your environment and life, you can promote harmony, health, and happiness. Learn to integrate and coordinate the relationships of the five colors (white, green, black, red, yellow) with the traditional Chinese theory of the five elements (metal, wood, water, fire, earth), and the theory of the five positions (east, west, south, north, center). Skilled application of these is useful in maintaining internal harmony within individuals and external harmony between them and nature.

364)   Learn to use color for harmonizing and balancing your life, health, and energy. Discover what colors make you feel inspired and uplifted.

365)   Ted Andrews, author of *How To Heal With Color* (Llewellyn Publications, 1993) writes, "When we are 'balanced,' we can more effectively rid ourselves of toxins, negativities and patterns that hinder our life processes. One way to achieve balance is through the use of color—a vibrational remedy that interacts with the human energy system to stabilize physical, emotional, mental, and spiritual conditions. You can learn to develop sensitivity to color vibrations, discover beneficial colors for many physical conditions, use colors to balance chakras (centers), rejuvenate your health and energy with color breaths, and tap into healing vibrations through colored lights, candles, and clothes." Use your intuition to learn what color combinations work best for you.

366)   L. Clark and Y. Martine, co-authors of *Health, Youth and Beauty Through Color Breathing* (Celestial Arts, 1976) write, "Some colors stimulate and others subdue. Colors have vibration; they possess qualities to ease pain and to change the human personality. Colors can be used to attract or repel..."

Dance & Music Therapies

Music therapy is used in many hospitals to help patients feel better by encouraging participation in enjoyable group activities. Playing musical instruments or singing can be uplifting, energizing, fun, and healing. Dance and movement may be incorporated into these programs.

367)   Talk to your doctor or therapist about getting into a music or dance therapy program, if you are interested in doing these activities.

368)   Listen to some soothing music at home. Pay attention to how the music makes you feel. Does it have a calming and relaxing effect on your body, mind, and emotions? Or, does it energize and uplift you?

369)   Listen to some enjoyable music and gently move or dance.

Hobbies

370)   Explore various hobbies that you may enjoy. Select one and become involved in it. Take a class or teach yourself about the hobby.

371)   Grow sprouts to use in making healthy salads or juices.

372) Grow an herb garden; use the herbs to prepare nutritious, tasty meals.

373) Get involved with an arts and crafts project. Eventually, you may be able to sell your handiwork. Make clay jewelry. Do flower arranging. Sew or do needlework. Work on your project a little each day. When it is completed, you will have something creative to wear, something to display in your home, or a lovely handmade gift for someone special.

374) Take photographs when you go on nature walks. Frame some of them for your home or give them as gifts. Put the rest of the pictures in a photo album, and add some pressed flowers from your walks.

375) Read uplifting books. Share them with friends and family members. If you have difficulty reading because of illness, find books with large print, read children's books, or enjoy books with beautiful photographs or drawings. If you are ill or disabled, you may qualify for free audio equipment and literature on tape. These may be available by mail through your public library. Or buy them at a discount book store.

376) Begin to collect stamps from around the world. Save stamps from the postcards and letters that you receive from friends and family members who travel to exotic places. Put these stamps in an album.

Chapter 8. Spiritual Health

"Not by might, nor by power, but by my spirit."
— Zechariah 4:6

Accessing our spiritual nature—through prayer, meditation, singing, chanting, yoga, community service, or by other means—can fill us with inspiration and strength, especially when living with chronic illness. Whether we call it "God," the "universe," a "higher power," or "life energy," spirituality is a powerful resource for healing. Developing spirituality for health does not have to be complex. It can be as simple as walking in a garden, sitting quietly and taking deep breaths, or enjoying a beautiful sunset. It doesn't even have to be "religious" in nature, if organized religion makes you uncomfortable. You don't have to believe in a particular religious practice to feel a sense of inner peace through a connection with your spirit. You need only to open your heart and mind to a higher power.

Larry Dossey, M.D. has written a number of spiritual and healing books, including *Healing Words: The power of prayer and the practice of medicine* (Harper San Francisco, 1993) and *Recovering The Soul, Meaning & Medicine*. He is co-chairman of the newly established Panel on Mind/Body Interventions, Office of Alternative Medicine, at the National Institutes of Health. After practicing medicine for many years, he was stunned to discover scientific evidence of the healing power of prayer. For ten years, he researched the relationship between prayer and healing. Dr. Dossey writes about the way prayer manifests in laboratory experiments, and he explores how modern physics may be compatible with these actions. He examines which methods of prayer show the greatest potential for healing and how one's innate temperament and personality affect prayer style. Addressing both patients and physicians, he presents evidence on how belief in a treatment can increase its effectiveness. He recommends more prayers of gratitude and fewer prayers of supplication. He says, "The world, at heart, is more glorious, benevolent, and friendlier than we have supposed."

"Prayer takes many forms," according to Dr. Dossey. "Many people follow the formalities of the great religions and pray explicitly for specific events to occur. Many people pray to a personal god or goddess, or to an impersonal universe. Others do not pray in any conventional sense, but live with a [deep inner] sense of the sacred. Theirs could be called a spirit of prayerfulness, a sense of simply being attuned or aligned with 'something higher.' Prayer tends to follow instructions laid down by the great religious traditions; prayerfulness does not. It is a feeling of unity with the All, rather than with specific leaders, traditions, or holy books. Some people pray for a specific outcome, to structure the future, to 'tell God what to do,' such as take [illness] away. Prayerfulness is accepting without being passive, it is grateful without giving up. It is being more willing to accept the rightness of whatever happens, even [illness]...If we allow ourselves to enter the quiet, still place of prayerfulness, we can understand the co-relationship of health and illness in the natural order." Prayerfulness helps us to understand and accept illness as a part of life.

"During illness," Dr. Dossey says, "we almost always want to do something about it, to take an antibiotic for a cold or rush to surgery. A certain amount of doing is always valuable and can even be lifesaving. But doing must be supplemented by *being*—looking inward, examining, focusing, wondering, asking. Being and doing are not incompatible; they can and should coexist. And for some people, the most effective way to reverse illness is to focus primarily on being."

Spirituality & Healing Tips

377)   Begin your day with a healing prayer.

378)   Dr. Gerald Jampolsky (author of *Love Is Letting Go Of Fear*, *Good Bye To Guilt*, *Teach Only Love*, *To Give Is To Receive*, and *18-Day Mini-Course on Healing Relationships*, etc.) says that his healing process starts at the beginning of the day. He devotes twenty minutes to silencing his mind and reminds himself what kind of day he wishes to experience—a day devoted to God. He is inspired by passages from *A Course In Miracles*.

379)   Pray. You may ask for strength, well-being, inner peace, healing, and prosperity. Be thankful for all of your blessings. Trust in life. Let go and let God help you heal your body and life. Be open to miracles.

380)   Attend a spiritual service that uplifts you and makes you feel good. Most services are open to everyone. Praying and singing in a group setting can be powerful, and make you feel less isolated. Or meet with a spiritual teacher for assistance with healing prayers.

381)   Write a prayer request and share it with close friends. Meet in a group, or with your family members, and pray together.

382)   Marianne Williamson, author of *A Return To Love: Reflections on the Principles of A Course in Miracles* (Harper Perennial, 1993), suggests that we consider miracles to be the power of the universe and they will be such for us. She writes, "The past is over…. The future can be reprogrammed [now]. We don't need another seminar, another degree, another lifetime, or anyone's approval in order for this to happen. All we have to do is ask for a miracle and allow it to happen, not resist it. There can be a new beginning, a new life, unlike the past." Our relationships shall be made new; our bodies shall be made new—not later, now. Nowhere, but here. Not through pain, but through peace.

Chapter 9. Healthy Relationships

Dr. John Gray (author of *What You Feel You Can Heal* and *Men Are From Mars, Women Are From Venus*) believes that "...An intimate relationship is the ideal setting for healing repressed feelings. When you find someone you feel safe with and loved by, all your repressed feelings begin to surface in an attempt to be healed." Through honest, loving relationships, you can learn to reduce tension between yourself and another person. A relationship can provide an opportunity to heal past wounds, freeing you to become a more loving and lovable person.

Chronic illnesses can strain relationships with family, partners, and friends, often to the breaking point. People may not understand your special needs. They may feel inadequate if they are unable to meet your needs. Do not feel guilty about being ill; it is *not* your fault. You may want to work with a supportive therapist to cope with relationship problems related to your illness. Consider joining a support group that encourages the participation of family members.

Friends and relatives may not always understand how your illness affects your life. Talk with them about what is happening to you and ask how they feel. If your appearance is not dramatically altered by your illness, people may assume that you are not seriously ill. They may expect you to recover quickly and resume your usual activities, which can put pressure on you. Or they may lose patience when your illness lingers. Illness can be devastating and recovery can be a slow, tedious process. Loved ones need to give and receive patience, understanding, and unconditional love—the basis of any healthy relationship. A stable, nurturing, and non-judgmental relationship can enhance your healing process.

If you are in an unsupportive relationship, you may decide that spending more time alone or with friends is better for your health. You may choose to end unhealthy relationships so that you can focus on building your health.

Nurture Your "Self"

383) Love and approve of yourself completely. This is essential to your well-being. It is well known that before you can experience loving another person, you must first love yourself. Therefore, release any doubts that you may have about feeling self-love. You deserve love.

384) Build and maintain your self-esteem and self-respect. Feel worthy of respect, affection, and appreciation.

385) Be willing to ask for help and be willing to receive it. Most people enjoy helping others and they find it rewarding.

386) Pamper yourself daily. Take a bath, wear comfortable clothes, drink herbal teas, meditate, listen to relaxing tapes, or eat healing foods.

387) Do what makes you feel special, important, and wonderful.

388) Have open, honest, loving communication with yourself and others.

389) Be true to yourself. Believe in yourself, focus on your feelings, and follow what is right for you.

390) Stay in touch with your feelings and express those feelings often. Believe that what you have to say is important.

391) Get a facial or give yourself one—using natural, hypoallergenic skin care products.

392) Make a list of your finest qualities and your achievements. Share them with a friend or mail them to yourself to read at a later time.

393) Make a list of what makes you feel warm and comfortable. Then do one thing on your list.

394)   Write yourself a love letter. Draw hearts on it or add colorful stickers. Write how much you mean to you. Include soothing and encouraging words that you would enjoy hearing from a loved one. Mail this letter to yourself or keep it in a special place. Read it again later.

395)   Write a list of things that you want and need. Begin to create those things, one at a time. For example, you need fresh air, clean water, healing foods, sunlight, hugs, love, laughter, and companionship. You may want to have a good conversation, read a good book, watch your favorite TV show, hear some lively music, get your work done, visit your doctor, or do errands. If you need help, ask for it.

396)   Think of people you admire. List the qualities they have that you appreciate and develop those qualities in yourself.

Healthy Communication

397)   Pay attention to how you feel and how you talk to yourself throughout each day. Build up a strong, healthy inner voice. Stop beating yourself up verbally. Have patience with yourself. Focus on what you do right and forgive yourself for any mistakes.

398)   Read *What To Say When You Talk To Yourself* by Shad Helmstetter, Ph.D. He writes, "During the first eighteen years of our lives, if we grew up in fairly average, reasonably positive homes, we were told 'No!,' or what we could *not* do, more than *148,000 times!....*" How often were you told "yes" or that you could do something? For most of us, the "yes's" we received did not balance out the "no's." You can reprogram your self-talk. Erase your old, negative, counterproductive programming and replace it with healthy, new, positive programming. Erase and replace. Dr. Helmstetter says it can be easy. You can learn to change your attitudes and behavior by changing your programming. By giving specific, productive new directions to your mind, you can make things work and keep them working.

399)   Nathaniel Branden, Ph.D., the author of several popular books on self-esteem, offers ways for you to live more consciously. He believes, "The only limits are imaginary." Tap into your true self to live more consciously. Identify areas in your life in which you operate with the most consciousness and then the least. Identify three areas to improve on with regard to your level of consciousness. Explore what seems most difficult about staying in high-level mental focus in these areas. Imagine your limitless potential. Say to yourself, "I have the power to grow and to participate in life more fully. I believe in me. I deserve happiness." Then work to create the power to achieve great things by using tools to raise your self-esteem. This is an act of mental participation. It takes time to raise your self-esteem; however, it will improve your relationships, your health, and your life.

400) Set healthy and appropriate boundaries with yourself and with others. Tell people what you need; don't make them guess. Say what you feel and think. Be open, honest, and direct. If someone is being verbally abusive, you must first recognize it to stop it. You can follow up with assertive behavior and set healthy limits by saying, "I feel uncomfortable when you talk to me like that. Please don't do it again."

401) Develop healthy communication skills. Read *Messages: The Communication Skills Book* by M. McKay, M. Davis, and P. Fanning (Oakland, CA: New Harbinger Publications, 1992, tenth printing). It covers basic skills (listening, self disclosure, expressing); advanced skills (body language, paralanguage, metamessages, hidden agendas, Transactional Analysis, clarifying language); conflict skills (assertiveness training, fair fighting, negotiation); social skills (prejudgment, making contact); family skills (sexual communication, parent effectiveness, family communications); and public skills (small groups, public speaking, and dealing with stage fright).

Healing Family Relationships

"Parents push our buttons because they installed them!"
(From the NBC TV hit series "Mad About You")

In ancient Hawaii, the "Kahuna" priests served various aspects of the gods. Several "schools" were devoted to different gods and to arts of life, including the healing arts. The power and effectiveness of this tradition is revealed by its survival today. Several dozen Hawaiian elders still carry on this traditional healing; their knowledge is precious to the culture. Their main focus is recognition of the human being as a spiritual entity, and they believe that healing happens through prayer. Each disease process is a function of spiritual disharmony. When disharmony is replaced by the peace of God's love, then the physical disease process is transformed into healing. After prayer, the next step is spiritual counseling called "Ho'oponopono" which means "to make right," to correct the individual's relationship with the Creator and family and friends, eliminating disease from family life. Ho'oponopono has been practiced for many centuries within Hawaiian families. It involves counseling sessions facilitated by a healer or respected elder family member. Relatives gather around a sick family member, talking out their differences with each other. Resolving family conflicts is an integral part of the healing process. (Excerpts from "Kahuna: Ancient Hawaiian Healers" by Steve Bogardus. *Venture Inward*, March/April, 1988).

Carolyn Foster, author of *The Family Patterns Workbook: Breaking Free from Your Past & Creating A Life Of Your Own* (Perigee Books, 1993), believes that many of our personal distresses and conflicts spring from our family legacy of thoughts, attitudes, and behaviors. Alcoholism, debilitating anger, and feelings about money, sex, and work—as well as our inner life and outer actions—can all be traced back to our family of origin. She teaches strategies for assessing family dynamics and strategies for making healthy lifestyle changes. She suggests that we each discover and evaluate our memories, feelings, and experiences through journal-writing to create a more conscious and healthy inner life. She also suggests that we uncover, slowly and carefully, the truths of our family experiences. Following exercises in her book or working with a therapist, can help you learn to appreciate the strength of your weaknesses. Then you can draw upon unrealized assets as you work to achieve healthy goals.

402) Establish healthy communication with your family, if possible. Encourage one another to feel good. Each person can learn to function well independently and as an important part of the group. Each person should be allowed to speak openly, directly, and honestly. Disagreements can be dealt with in constructive ways. Problems or bad feelings can be overcome by working together to find resolutions.

403) Get family therapy; it may be beneficial for coping with your illness.

404) List loving qualities about family members and share it with them.

405) Mother Teresa said, "We must bring that presence of God into our families. And how do we do that? By praying."

A Nurturing Love Life

406) Make a list of qualities that you are looking for in a loving relationship. After writing what you want, make a list of what you do not want. List what you will not tolerate (such as someone who drinks too much, smokes, or who is verbally abusive). Your lists will help you clarify the person you are looking for. Make this an enjoyable, ongoing exercise. When you find someone interesting, check your list and decide if the person has compatible qualities.

407) Believe that you are deserving of a loving partner. Know you deserve unconditional love, a nurturing partner, acceptance, understanding, compassion, and passion. Begin by loving yourself in these ways.

408)   When you are ill, don't upset yourself by comparing your life to your partner's. Tell yourself that your life is just as important—even if for now you have to spend many days resting in bed. It is your job to rest and get well. A loving partner will respect and support your needs.

409)   Set healthy limits with your partner. Rebecca Sydnor, author of *Making Love Happen* (Avon Books, 1989), writes: "The right way to set limits is: from the beginning, consistently, in a calm and straightforward manner, without feeling guilty. The wrong way to set limits is: inconsistently, only in a crisis, hysterically, and while feeling guilty." The author teaches a woman to: find the man of her dreams, choose from dozens of eligible men, use her heart and her head to recognize the best prospects, avoid wasting time on dead-end relationships, and to feel confident.

410)   Join Codependents Anonymous, a 12-Step healing/recovery program, if you have difficulty with intimacy, trust, jealousy, etc. Read Melody Beattie's books on healing/recovery: *Codependent No More* (Harper & Row, 1987); *Beyond Codenpendency* (Harper & Row, 1989); and *Codependents' Guide To The Twelve Steps* (Simon & Schuster, 1990).

Healthy Friendships & A Healthy Social Life

411)   Focus on improving the quality, not the quantity, of your friendships. Healthy friendships have these essential qualities: mutual respect and admiration, openness, honesty, trust, integrity, and cooperation. There is a balance of giving and receiving. Trust is built as friends consistently say what they mean and mean what they say. Good friends are loving, loyal, supportive, kind, patient, and understanding. Do not accept friendships that are negative, draining, or abusive.

412)   Always set healthy limits with yourself and others. Tell people what you need, especially concerning your health. Work to meet those needs.

413)   Socialize only when you feel up to it. Even if you have made plans, do not feel obligated to go out when you are too tired or ill. Friends should understand if you have to cancel plans because of illness. Explain that you need time for resting and healing. Offer to reschedule your plans when you feel stronger and ready to socialize. Pacing yourself is essential to healing and recovery. Do not compare what others are doing in their lives to what you are doing. Instead, keep your focus on your healing efforts and on your life. Know that you are a person of value to yourself, to your loved ones, and to society.

Chapter 10. Prosperity & Creating The Right Livelihood

Developing the right attitude about money is a good way to improve your financial situation. Earning money and staying productive, even when dealing with illness, requires setting realistic goals and doing things as your energy allows.

Marianne Williamson, author of A *Return To Love* (based on the principles of *A Course in Miracles*) suggests asking the Holy Spirit to remove any obstacles to receiving money. Obstacles can take the form of negative thinking, such as 'money is impure' or 'having money means we're greedy." Some people may think that "Money is the root of all evil." There is nothing wrong with having money or being prosperous. We can choose to think of money in a positive light, such as: "When we have more money, we can help others and help heal the world."

Joe Dominquez and Vicki Robin, authors of *Your Money or Your Life: Transforming Your Relationship with Money and Achieving Financial Independence*, write: "Money is morally neutral. Money isn't evil, even though some people may choose to do evil things with it." They suggest ways to save money: pay off your credit cards; eliminate all but one credit card for emergencies and stop paying unnecessary annual fees; don't bounce checks; and try to pay cash for all purchases, even major ones. You can also follow their checklist before spending money: don't shop compulsively; live within your means; take care of what you have; wear it out; do it yourself; anticipate your needs; research value, quality, durability, and multiple use; get it for less; and buy used goods.

They recommend other financial tips regarding health care. As medical costs are rising, trying to improve your health is good for your pocketbook as well as your body. Health care begins at home. Stop smoking and limit drinking alcohol. Eat healthy foods. Get as much exercise as your energy permits. To cut medical expenses: get proper medical insurance; and comparison-shop for prescription drugs, blood tests, X-rays, and other procedures. Many doctors can see patients at different hospitals. Find out which hospital would be least expensive for you.

Prosperous Thinking

In her book, *The Dynamic Laws of Prosperity*, Catherine Ponder explores the power of prosperous thinking. An inspirational author of more than a dozen books, she is a minister of the nondenominational Unity faith, serving in Unity churches since 1956. She also heads a global ministry in Palm Desert, California. She writes, "You are prosperous to the degree that you are experiencing peace, health, and plenty in your world. [Prosperous thinking] gives you the power to make your dreams come true, whether those dreams are concerned with better health, increased financial success, a happier personal life, more education and travel, or a deeper spiritual life." Such thinking can create inner peace, self-confidence, happiness, security, and stability. After being widowed, Catherine Ponder was left with a small son to raise. She had no training for work and no income. After experiencing depression, ill health, loneliness, financial lack, and a sense of complete failure, she decided that she had to succeed for her son's sake and her own. When she was at her lowest point emotionally, physically, and financially, she learned about the "power of thought as an instrument for success or failure." She realized that "failure is basically the result of failure thinking," and that "the right use of her mind could become the key to a healthy, happy, and prosperous life." When she grasped these secrets for success, her life began to change. She began sharing her experiences and counseling others.

After observing how thinking affects health directly, she wrote, "Many people who are in poor health, due to worry over financial problems, find it almost uncanny how fast their health improves as their financial situation improves. Prosperous thinking is victorious, harmonious, uplifted thinking." A prosperous thinker knows how to become free of hostilities, resentments, criticisms, and irritations—and works toward achieving balanced, normal thinking which reflects a will to win. Often depression and a feeling of defeat can cause ill health. To overcome feeling hopeless, helpless, and defeated, and to adopt a winning attitude, she suggests repeating these words: "Divine love and wisdom go before me, making easy and successful my way.... The divine solution now quickly and easily appears. I am now guided, healed, prospered, and blessed."

"Prosperity is our divine heritage, " Catherine Ponder believes. "As you study the lives and experiences of prosperous-minded people, you will find that they have a friendly attitude toward money. Money is wonderful because it is divine substance and money is good when rightly used."

Prosperity Principles

Sharon Connors, M.A., minister of Unity Church in San Francisco, suggests using these twelve "prosperity principles" (universal laws of prosperity) often:

414) Establish order in your life, both outside and inside. For example, balance your checkbook, do your taxes, or organize your paperwork. Organizing on the outside helps you feel more organized inside. Do one thing each day to establish order. By developing spirituality, your life can be different and better. Putting God first on an emotional level can get you on track with "internal" order. God can be in your life every day, not just on Sundays. Talk to God, pray, and meditate.

415) Forgive yourself and others. When you don't forgive, you may feel a wall of separation. Even though some things are difficult to forgive, you can send love to anyone with whom you're having difficulty. Ask God to forgive through you.

416)   Develop a faith-building program. Take steps each day to establish faith in your life. Take risks and put God first. For example, say hello to someone who seems unhappy.

417)   Tithe. Give a percentage of your income to wherever you get spiritual nourishment.

418)   View God as your partner and employer. Dedicate yourself to God, in your business and in everything you do. Make God your employer. You do the work and God handles the rest.

419)   Nourish yourself—your spirit, soul, and body—on a daily basis. Prayer in groups is powerful. Nurturing your soul nurtures your body. Getting enough exercise, eating a healthy diet, and having a positive attitude are ways to nourish yourself.

420)   Accept yourself with compassion so that you are free to change.

421)   Develop a "give" attitude and dedicate all that you do to God. Create mutual support in your life. Listen to others and have them listen to you, giving each other your full attention.

422)   Be willing to change, or be willing to be willing. Set the right attitude. Develop "indestructible" inner strength.

423)   Don't worry about controlling everything. "Let go and let God."

424)   Develop a gratitude litany and an attitude of gratitude. There is so much to be grateful for in life—such as walks, talks, the beauty of nature, and sharing hugs. Say to yourself, "I have a gratitude attitude. My life is a miracle of rich rewards and happiness."

425)   Get clear on your desires and purposes. Work with the Divine idea of love. There's nothing love can't do.

Learn Marketable Skills

426)   If you feel well enough to work part-time on a flexible schedule, talk to your doctor or a social worker about finding a rehabilitation program in order to learn some new job skills. Choose an area that will be of interest to you—and one that involves activities that are not too stressful or physically unhealthy. Or take classes that offer job training in computers and other marketable areas.

Pursue A Degree

427) Consider taking classes part-time or pursuing a certificate or degree. Meet with a school counselor and discuss possible programs. If you need financial help, find out about the school's financial aid policies. Many colleges have special services for disabled students. If it is difficult for you to take notes, get someone to attend your classes and take notes for you. Or get permission to tape record a teacher's lecture.

428) Consider taking courses through the Mind Extension University ® (ME/U™). You may contact them for a catalog. Call: 1-800-777-MIND. Or write: ME/U, 9697 East Mineral Ave., P.O. Box 6612, Englewood, Colorado 80155-6612. The ME/U is the nation's only cable television channel that is exclusively dedicated to educational programming. ME/U delivers a college campus right to your home or workplace. It unites students and universities. They offer opportunities to take college courses, or earn a graduate or undergraduate degree from more than 25 regionally accredited universities. ME/U Programming also includes non-credit courses and certificate programs for career advancement and personal enrichment—such as languages, computer training, and business. This unique service offers you one-stop enrollment, removing all obstacles of returning to college.

Alternative Ways To Earn Money / Self-Employment

Working at home can be an excellent way to continue earning some money when you are chronically ill. There are many advantages to creating a home-based business—that's why it has become so popular. First, you have greater freedom and flexibility because you can usually set your own hours and schedule your own appointments. That way you can work a few hours, rest, see your doctor, go for a walk, call a friend, spend more time with your children, and go back to work when you're ready—or you can take the rest of the afternoon off if you're too ill or tired. Setting your own schedule provides a perfect opportunity to pace yourself, based on your energy level and how you feel during each day. To find out about additional tax advantages to working at home, consult an accountant.

Developing your own business can allow you to have more creative control—from the work you choose to do to how you choose to do your work. When choosing a business, it helps to know yourself, your strengths, and your limitations. It is essential to research every aspect of your potential new business. Having your own business also allows you to choose the type of people you deal with on a regular basis. Working on your own can eliminate the stress of "office politics" or personality conflicts. Choose to work with people who are generally optimistic, encouraging, and supportive. Rather than taking on partnerships, consider building your own business and encouraging others to do the same.

429)   Develop a small business at home one step at a time—one that will be enjoyable and creative for you, and one that will not be too stressful.

430)   Consult with organizations such as the Small Business Association (SBA), Service Corps of Retired Executives (SCORE), or the American Association of Retired Persons (AARP). For more information on AARP, call (202) 434-2277 in Washington, D.C.

431)   Take small business classes at a community college or university. Many adult education classes are free or low cost. Or consider applying for a degree program in business or a creative field of interest (computers, art, music, English, etc.). After meeting people with similar interests, you can set up a support network to help you achieve your educational and business goals.

432)   Consult with several experts or small business owners in your field of interest for objective advice. Ask if they are willing to discuss their field. Find out what they enjoy most about their work. Ask about the most challenging and most rewarding aspects of their businesses.

433)   If you have experience in a particular field, consider becoming a business consultant.

434)   "Brainstorm" with others about producing and marketing your ideas, products, or services. However, be cautious about giving your ideas away and about forming partnerships. To prevent problems or disagreements that may arise with partners, it may be best to work with others on a freelance basis. As your business expands, you may hire temporary help through a reputable agency, or you may hire consultants/independent contractors who are recommended to you. Or you can hire additional help on a per-project basis. Consult a lawyer before you sign a contract.

435)   Make your home office environment pleasant and comfortable. Consider using full-spectrum light bulbs. Choose your favorite colors when designing and decorating your office. Houseplants add warmth and beauty to a room, and some plants may help to detoxify the air. You can usually control noise and stress in your own office. Listening to soft music while you work can be relaxing.

436)   Working at home makes commuting a breeze. Commuting from your bedroom down the hallway to your office may take only seconds. You can save your own energy and energy on gas for your car, while helping the environment by not polluting the air. You usually have more control over air quality and temperature in your own office. You can open a window and let in fresh air and sunlight. (When working for someone else, you may be exposed to a flu virus or cigarette smoke.)

437)   You save time and money by not commuting to work. Put these valuable "savings" into creatively developing your own business— one that you find pleasurable and meaningful.

438)   Learn to work in a productive, efficient, and effective manner. It is essential to streamline your life when living with a chronic illness.

439)   Be sure to set up a business plan and structure that is right for you, one that is appropriate for your specific health requirements. The most important thing is to pace yourself by paying close attention to how you feel. Don't forget that you can take frequent breaks whenever you need to because you're the boss!

440)   Find out about getting state, federal, or private disability benefits if or whenever you are too ill to work.

441)   If you work for an employer, try to arrange to do your work (or, at least, some of your work) at home by tele-commuting via computer, telephone, and a fax. This arrangement is becoming more popular.

442)   Change jobs or careers if you need to work in a less stressful environment. Or find creative ways to supplement your income.

443)   *The Best Home Businesses For The '90s: The Inside Information You Need To Know To Select A Home-Based Business That's Right For You*, by Paul and Sarah Edwards (the "Self-Employment Experts"), profiles 70 top businesses. How each business works and what skills can help, how much you can earn, how much it costs to get started, where to begin, how to get customers, what you can charge for your product or service, and much more. (N.Y.: G. P. Putnam's Sons, 1991.)

444)   Turn one of your hobbies into a small business. Some of America's most successful companies started this way: Laurel Burch, the jewelry designer, and Mrs. Fields, the cookie maker, are excellent examples. It is much easier to work when you love what you're doing.

445)   Sell things that you no longer need at flea markets or garage sales.

446)   If you have a chronic illness but are still able to work for an employer, consider applying for disability insurance (either through your employer or a private policy, which is usually more expensive).

447)   Read *Working From Home: Everything You Need To Know About Living & Working Under The Same Roof* by Paul and Sara Edwards.

448)   Barter for goods and/or services with friends or your support group.

449)   Apply for a government rehabilitation or an unemployment program to help further your education or to find a job that you can handle.

450)   Lynie Arden, author of *The Work-At-Home Sourcebook*, lists over 1,000 companies by state that use qualified home workers. Categories include opportunities in crafts and home-based computer work. Specifics are listed, such as pay scale and work requirements.

451)   Take a self-employment class or seminar. Talk to a business consultant or an accountant about how to set up an accounting system and how to handle your tax forms. Learn which tax deductions apply to your home-based business.

452)   Barbara Brabec, author of *Homemade Money: The Definitive Guide to Success*, gives practical, expert advice on: getting started; selecting the right home business and avoiding the wrong ones; and planning for profits and success. This A to Z course in business basics provides information on selling direct and selling to wholesale markets. It lists strategies for diversification and expansion, and it includes more than 500 valuable information-by-mail resources.

453)   Avid readers may decide to make money by reading books. One reference is: *Make Money Reading Books: How to Start and Operate Your Own Home-based Freelance Reading Service* by Bruce Fife (Distributed by Ingram, 1993). This book is for people who want to use English skills for a livelihood. It explores "reading" jobs such as: being a reading aide in schools; reviewing; proofreading; or becoming a literary agent or indexer. The author cautions about some reading scams. For example, be wary if you are asked to pay money up front.

454)   Talk to a consultant, or someone working in your field, about what to charge for your products or services. Learn what your time, skills, and knowledge are worth, and set appropriate fees. Learn to handle expenses and collect fees. Learn to avoid problems, such as disputes about costs. Write a proposal or contract and get the client's approval before starting the work. You may ask for partial payment upfront.

455)   Consider setting up a home-based typing business. Potential clients may be in these areas: academic, medical, business, legal, or media.

456)   Susan Ratliff is a successful weekend entrepreneur and author of *How To Be A Weekend Entrepreneur: Making Money at Craft Fairs & Trade Shows* (Login, 1994). The book offers tips for people needing additional income. It tells how to set up and run a weekend business. It lists craft fairs, trade shows, swap meets, sources, and supplies.

457)   Call 1-800-421-2300 for a free catalog from *Entrepreneur* magazine called, "The Small Business Development Catalog." It provides 180 small business start-up guides, about 200 pages each, outlining various potential business opportunities for you.

Community Service / Volunteer Work

Some people who live with illness may still have energy for part-time volunteer work. Volunteering can provide opportunities for keeping active and productive. When illness causes depression, isolation, or low self-esteem because of inactivity, helping others is an effective way to help yourself feel better. It is also a good way to meet people. Sharing your time, talents, and enthusiasm is rewarding. Making a meaningful contribution to others' lives enriches your own life. For more information, read *Stand Up and Be Counted: The Volunteer Resource Book* by Judy Knipe (Simon & Schuster, 1992). It has hundreds of unique and rewarding ideas for individuals, families, businesses, schools, and churches.

458)   A wide range of volunteer work is available. Volunteers are welcome in organizations, libraries, churches, schools, and hospitals. Some organizations provide services for underprivileged children, single parents, the mentally or physically challenged, or disabled seniors. You may choose to tutor children or foreign students, mentor a teen or young adult, share your travel experiences by giving slideshows, tell stories, sing, or play an instrument. Many educational programs may need your help to teach reading, writing, math, or computer skills. Learn valuable job skills or get college credit for your work.

459)   Share your artistic talents or hobbies by teaching drawing, painting, sewing, photography, woodworking, or music.

460)   Volunteers are always needed to help raise funds for charities. Much of this work can be done by telephone.

461)   What you would most enjoy doing? How can this benefit others?

462)   Some agencies list and refer people to nonprofit organizations which need volunteers. They can match your interests and skills to an organization in your area. Contact your librarian for information.

Chapter 11. Developing An Effective Support Network

Being ill can cause you to feel a wide range of emotions, including loneliness, discouragement, or fear. Illness can also cause psychological problems, such as stress, anxiety, or depression. You may want to seek professional help to cope with any emotional issues or to change any negative thought patterns. Working with a compassionate therapist, or joining a support group, may help you to develop inner strength for coping and inner peace for healing. Nurturing friendships can also be a source of great comfort and encouragement. Be sure to structure your life, especially your social life, according to how you feel.

Note: If you ever feel severely depressed, hopeless, or in despair, contact your doctor, therapist, health care provider, social worker, a hotline service, minister, spiritual counselor, family member, or a friend. Call 911 for emergencies. Find support and a safe haven when you need help.

463)   Find self-nurturing activities to increase self-awareness, cultivate a sense of security, and develop self-love and appreciation.

464)   Learn to cope with isolation by getting more involved with your healing program, by taking classes, or developing hobbies. Begin to enjoy your time alone. View your time alone as an opportunity for you to relax, rest, rejuvenate, take a long bath, read, write, exercise, pray, or meditate. Free from distractions, these activities can be enlightening and healing.

465)   When you feel more energetic, spend time socializing. Invite a loved one over for a pot luck meal. Go for a walk together. Or see a movie.

466)   Attending a place of worship and praying in a group can help you to feel a sense of community, support, and strength.

467)   Get involved with a group activity or a community service project, one that isn't too stressful or time-consuming.

468)   Develop a nurturing romantic relationship. A loving partner can offer tender loving care, affection, and warm companionship.

469)   Keep a phone-buddy list handy on the refrigerator door or near the telephone. Call someone on that list when you feel sad, lonely, depressed, or in need of help.

470)   Make a help-line list of people you can count on in times of need. List people from your support group, loving friends, a supportive counselor, a caring minister, your doctor, or anyone who can be there when you need help or when you need encouragement. Choose people who are caring and uplifting, people who are willing and able to offer you help and reassurance when you need it. Choose compassionate people who are good listeners, and those who have strength and patience. You can offer them support in return when they need it.

471)   While it may feel a little uncomfortable to reach out for help, do not let that stop you. Caring people are more than happy to be there for you. They will want to share their strength, hope, and optimism because it is rewarding to help others.

472)   As you learn to listen more carefully to your thoughts, feelings, and body, you will know when you need to reach out for help. Reaching out for help when you need it is actually a loving thing to do for yourself. It supports your health care program. Fortunately, we live in a society where helpful and supportive people and organizations are usually available. Don't be shy about asking for help.

473)   Your well-being is always important. For help or for any emergencies, call 911, Suicide Prevention, or your local hospital. Don't go without help. There are places for you to turn and people who will care.

Caregivers

474)   If you are a caregiver, learn the most effective ways to support others, while finding the right support for yourself. Encourage someone who is ill to make healthier lifestyle choices. Set a positive example. Offer positive feedback and encouragement; do not judge or criticize. Read *Giving Comfort: What You Can Do When Someone You Love Is Ill* by L. B. Milstein (Penguin Books, 1994).

475)   *Care Pooling: How to Get the Help You Need to Care for the Ones You Love* (Berrett-Koehler Publishers, 1993) by Paula C. Lowe offers ways for caregivers to get more help and support. She provides tools for: identifying potential "carepoolers" (a network of support), understanding why it is hard to ask for help, initiating carepooling relationships, creating written guidelines, resolving conflicts among carepoolers, and hiring a shared care provider.

476)   Melvin Pohl, M.D. and Deniston J. Kay, Ph.D., authors of *Staying Sane: When You Care For Someone With Chronic Illness* (Health Communications, 1993), list creative ideas and activities to brighten your day and keep your spirits up. The compassionate authors offer ways to care for loved ones, while taking care of your own needs.

Their upbeat, motivational approach lightens the heavy burden of caregiving, showing how to care for others without losing yourself. If you are the wife, husband, family member, nurse, counselor, friend, or lover of someone who is chronically ill, you need support.

477)   In her book, *Caring for the Caregiver: A Nurse's Journey to Health and Inner Peace* (Happy Talk Books, 1993), Roberta M. Jarrett provides honest and insightful caregiving tips on keeping mentally, physically, and emotionally fit while taking care of others.

478)   People with chronic illness need patience, understanding, respect, and love from their caregivers. And caregivers certainly need the same consideration and respect. By working together and communicating openly and honestly, everyone will feel better.

479)   Doctors and caregivers can help support the family members of chronically-ill patients by providing honest and clear information. Read *Taking Care Of Your Aging Family Members* by N.R. Hooyman and W. Lustbader (New York: The Free Press, 1986).

Chapter 12. Creating Optimism & A Bright Future

Christopher Peterson and Lisa M. Bossio, co-authors of *Health and Optimism* (The Free Press, 1991), studied and wrote about how psychological states affect physical health. They examined healthy and unhealthy aspects of lifestyles of individuals and of whole communities. Their book explores and establishes the link between health and optimism.

Surprisingly, many people experience positive outcomes from learning to adjust to their illnesses. They develop healthier attitudes and healthier lifestyles. Some people have become stronger after making more appropriate health choices. Many people have improved their relationships by being more open and honest.

Lifestyle Options To Consider For Coping With Illness

480) **Lifestyle**. I now create a simpler, more balanced, and peaceful lifestyle. I am more committed to taking better care of myself. I am more in tune with my thoughts, feelings, and body. I rest and relax, according to my health needs.

481) **Home**. I make my home a safer and healthier environment. I keep my home clean, neat, and organized—and I get help if necessary.

482) **Exercise**. Based on my doctor's advice, I set up an appropriate exercise program. I become involved with more health-promoting activities and do them with my family and friends.

483) **Nutrition**. I reduce my intake of fats, sugar, and junk food. I purchase and eat more nutritious foods. I stop unhealthy habits. I drink less alcohol and less caffeine. I quit smoking and do not abuse drugs.

484) **Holistic healing**. I regularly practice meditation, yoga, Qi Gong self-massage, visualization, or other forms of stress reduction.

485) **Pleasure**. I incorporate more enjoyable activities into my life. I do things that I have always dreamed of doing. I explore new places— such as museums, art galleries, beaches, and parks. I get involved with more creative projects and hobbies.

486) **Relationships.** I improve my relationships by communicating more openly and honestly. I spend more quality time with my loved ones. I spend time with people who are loving, supportive, fun, and uplifting. I let go of people who are abusive, unsupportive, or unhealthy. I am more selective about my social activities. I go out with people only when I feel up to it—and only when I have the time and energy.

487) **Love and Romance**. I enjoy more romantic times with my mate. I write letters, expressing and clarifying my thoughts, desires, and feelings. We learn to give and receive massages. We enjoy candlelight dinners. We go for long nature walks. We take vacations whenever possible. We spend more time being loving, intimate, and peaceful.

488) **Support**. I am not shy about asking for help when I need it. I reciprocate support whenever I can. I participate in a support group and find new strength. I get professional help from a caring therapist.

489) **Time Management**. I reset my priorities, according to my health needs and values. I reschedule appointments whenever I feel too ill or low on energy. I spend more time nurturing myself and others.

490) **Work**. I alter my work schedule or change jobs if necessary to cope with my illness. I develop a home-based business, which is more suited to my needs and talents—such as writing, arts, crafts, or music. I make my work environment healthier and safer, and less stressful.

491) **Education and Research**. I read books that enhance my life and lift my spirit. I learn about alternative healing practices and methods. I attend health classes to learn more about my illness. I learn new marketable skills. I take a computer class and further my knowledge and enhance my skills. I return to school part-time to earn a degree. I take creative classes, such as art or music, for fun and enjoyment.

492) **Entertainment**. I enjoy watching films, videos, or television programs of special interest. I watch travel videos and discover exciting and exotic places. I read about other places or cultures.

493) **Feelings**. I work through and release regrets, guilt, pain, and anger. Releasing anger gives me more energy. I forgive myself and others.

494) **Self-esteem**. I say kind and loving things to myself. I appreciate my accomplishments. I stop being critical of myself. I understand my limitations and work around them. I value and respect myself.

495) **Healing Attitudes**. I learn to love myself unconditionally. I let go of judging myself and others. I have more patience. I become more open-minded. I develop trust in myself and others. I strive to see the basic good in other people and in the world. I accept reality and do not deny the truth. I have faith that my life is getting better every day. I allow other people to have their own views, opinions, and feelings. I let go of trying to change others. Instead, I work to change myself.

496) Journal Writing. I keep a health care journal or record of my healing progress, dreams, support group experiences, or health care tips.

497) Volunteering. I spend a little time each week, or each month, helping, teaching, or supporting others who are ill or disabled. I reach out to others by smiling, joking, sharing, caring, and by being there.

498) Environmental Health. I learn and do all that I can to promote the health of the planet. I do my part to contribute to cleaning up the environment and to making the world a healthier and safer place.

499) Spirituality. I pray for spiritual healing within myself and my home. I pray for peace in our community, our country, and our world.

500) A Bright Outlook. I keep a list of people, places, and things for which I am most grateful. I deeply appreciate my life's miracles, both large and small. I live my life to the fullest each day. I keep a list of places that I want to explore and things that I want to do when I have the time and energy. I maintain a positive attitude and a good sense of humor. I feel good about myself. I believe in my body's ability to heal and be well. I think optimistically about my life and my future.

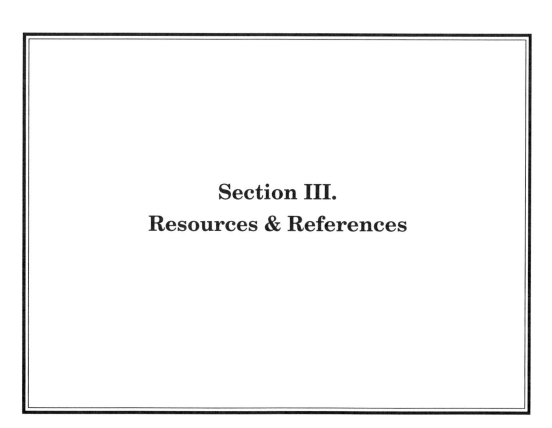

Section III.
Resources & References

Chapter 13. Resources For Help & Information

Computer databases, reference materials, books, magazines, professional journals, pamphlets, brochures, audio and video tapes, and many other resources are available in most libraries, colleges, universities, hospitals, and clinics. Don't be shy about asking for help with finding information. Most people will be happy to share their knowledge, references, contacts, and ideas with you.

Computer Databases & Networks

If you own a computer and a modem, or if you are able to use a computer in a public library or university, you can access a wide range of databases and bulletin boards. These offer information on most illnesses, including recommended treatments and the latest research. Computers can direct you to more contacts and provide you with more data than you can possibly ever use in this lifetime. They can help you find support groups, doctors, therapists, hotline services, hospitals, agencies, programs, and other resources; or they can help you access thousands of books and countless journal, magazine, and newspaper articles.

People can assist and encourage each other as they travel together on the "information highway." Whether they live in the same town, another state, or another country, people can explore the world of computers—while sharing support and information. Computers help people to overcome feelings of isolation, which is a common problem when dealing with illness. And computers can help people to establish local, national, and global health network communities.

Note: If you have no idea how to use computer equipment, don't let that scare or stop you. Ask a friend or a librarian for assistance. Or take a beginning computer class. Some knowledge and skill are required to navigate your way along the electronic highway, and this may present a challenge to the beginner. Many books and resource guides are available on this subject.

Ask a friend or a librarian for help to show you how to access and use computer databases and bulletin boards. Learn how to find information about your illness. And learn to find and communicate with other people who have the same illness as you do. Then begin to share tips, information, research, experiences, referrals, or ideas. Develop new contacts for friendship and support. Caution: Be careful about believing everything you read. And be cautious about any requests for money. While computers can provide endless possibilities for help and support, they may also provide opportunities for abuse. Don't allow anyone to take advantage of you or your situation. Use good common sense and check things out. Contact organizations, such as the Better Business Bureau, before getting involved with a "business opportunity." Get to know someone through the computer over a period of time before agreeing to meet him or her in person.

Don't be afraid to explore the world of computers, if you haven't already. These powerful tools can inform you, while enhancing your business, communication, hobbies, education, and health care options. They can provide you with endless hours of fun and entertainment. Sometimes, they even help to save lives! Take advantage of what information you can find and use on a computer, and enjoy the learning process. Who knows where computers may lead you? Chances are they will open new doors and help you to get on a healthy, new track. Hopefully, they will lead you to useful information and help you to establish a support network! Note: If you are often unable to leave your bed, borrow a laptop computer from a friend or a family member if possible. Ask them to teach you how to use it. Or just enjoy playing some computer games.

Medical CD-ROMs (Computer Software)

Medical computer programs offer a wide range of invaluable health care information—from basic anatomy to harmful drug interactions. Prices may range from $50 to $100 each.

Some CD-ROM Health Guides:
Mayo Clinic Family Health Book: The Ultimate Interactive Guide to Health (IVI Publishing, Inc.). The disc explains basic anatomy and diseases, illustrates procedures, and provides first aid and safety tips.

Dr. Schueler's Home Medical Advisor Pro (Pixel Perfect). This disc helps users identify symptoms of illnesses, it lists poisons and what to do if ingested, and it helps patients to analyze and avoid drug interactions.

The Family Doctor (Creative Multimedia). Answers the most commonly asked questions on more than 280 conditions.

HealthDesk 1.2 (HealthDesk Corp.). Helps you track medical costs, conditions, vaccinations, and doctor and hospital visits. Helps you count calories, keep track of weight loss or gain, monitor blood pressure, and keep a log of exercise routines. Offers helpful hints about various health issues.

Medical Matters (Parsons Technology). Health journal and reference tool. Medicare information. Provides the names, addresses, and phone numbers of 500 health and medical agencies.

Health Soft Complete Guide to Symptoms, Illness, and Surgery (Great Bear Technology). Graphics show various surgical procedures. Helps users identify diseases associated with symptoms and vice versa.

Some CD-ROM Anatomy Programs:
3-D Body Adventure (Knowledge Adventure)
Bodyworks Voyager (Software Marketing Corp.)
A.D.A.M.: The Inside Story (A.D.A.M. Software)
Bodyworks 3.0 (Software Marketing Corp.) Shows 3-D rotating views of various body parts, and information on fitness and common illnesses.

Some CD-ROM Drug Guides:

PharmAssist (Software Marketing Corp.) Quick, easy-to-understand
information on drugs, ranging from allergy pills to painkillers. Hundreds of
color images help user identify drugs by size, shape, and color. A section on
administering and taking prescription and non-prescription drugs, and a drug
interaction section.

**Mayo Family Pharmacist: Your Ultimate Guide to Medications, Early
Detection, and First Aid** (IVI Publishing)

HealthSoft Complete Guide to Prescription & Non-Prescription Drugs
(Great Bear Technology).

Computer On-Line Services

Using an on-line database can be your most helpful advisor at times. Databases
and on-line services can allow you to access information on thousands of subjects.
There are unlimited medical and health care information and services. **Women's
Wire** specializes in women's health issues. **Sapient Health Network** offers
an information service for patients, many of whom are chronically or terminally
ill. Healthcare consumers can receive specific information which can enable
them to better manage and control their situations. Write to: Sapient Health
Network, 10 NW 10th Avenue, Suite 430, Portland, OR 97209; call (800) 353-
1231; or check out their web site at: www.shn.net.

Commercial Computer On-Line Services

Most of these computer services offer free hours of use with initial subscription. They charge monthly fees, plus hourly rates beyond the minimum. To order the *On-Line Access* (a magazine of databases), call: (312) 755-9100 in Chicago, IL.

Service	Telephone
Microsoft Network	(800) 386-5550
America Online	(800) 827-6364
CompuServe	(800) 848-8199

(Includes access to research-based information and a
  large support network for chronic illness.)

GEnie	(800) 638-9636

(Medical round table and various medical products.)

Prodigy	(800) PRODIGY (822-6922)

General Medical Resources

Visit health information services and libraries to research your illness. University medical schools and most hospitals have health resource centers. Such resource centers have medical journals, books, and computer databases. If you need help using a computer, ask someone at the information desk for assistance. To begin your computer search, select categories or key phrases relating to your particular illness. Enter each category or phrase into the computer, one at a time. You may usually print out information to take with you.

Call the National Institutes of Health (NIH) in Bethesda, Maryland for information about your illness. Telephone: (301) 496-4000.

Call the Centers For Disease Control (CDC) in Atlanta, Georgia for information about your illness. Telephone: (404) 332-4555.

The Medical Information Line by Strategic System, Inc. Call: 1-900-230-4800. For up to date, confidential, reliable information on over 300 pre-recorded topics. This health education material is reviewed favorably by the American Academy of Family Physicians Foundation. ($1.95 per minute. Topics average 5 minutes.)

Wear a Medic Alert ID. For information, call: 1-800-432-5378.

Sources For General Research

Libraries. Begin your search for more information on this subject at your local library, which has a wealth of resources. Librarians are your best source of help. You may ask them for assistance, for specific information, and for suggestions on where to find references. Some resources are listed below.

Computer/CD ROM Searches/On-Line Databases. Most major libraries have computer on-line services. This new technology may be the most useful for research regarding your illness. CD-ROM offers comprehensive information on your topic. Computer searches will help you locate a wide range of materials. Many databases are available. You may ask your librarian how to use the computer system. Computers can open a world of ideas, support, and information.

Subject Guide to Books in Print. R. R. Bowker Company, New York. Over 300,000 books by American publishers are listed alphabetically by subject. There are over 60,000 subject headings with over 50,000 cross references.

Subject Guide to Forthcoming Books. R. R. Bowker Company, New York. This guide lists books that will be published within the next five months.

Paperbound Books in Print. R. R. Bowker Company, New York. Over 100,000 titles are listed by subject, author, and title.

Books in Print. R. R. Bowker Company, New York. This four-volume guide contains over 400,000 books in print in the U.S. Two volumes contain alphabetical listings by author, and two offer a listing of available books by title.

Publishers Trade List Annual. R. R. Bowker Co. N.Y. Lists publishers' catalogs, providing all of the titles available from each publisher; arranged alphabetically by publisher. It is useful when a publisher has a number of titles on a particular subject. This manual can save you time if you're trying to find several books on the same subject.

The Cumulative Book Index. H. H. Wilson Company, Bronx, New York. This index lists all books published from 1928 to the present that are still in print. It includes the price of each book and the publisher's address.

Director of Special Libraries and Information Centers. Gale Research, Detroit, Michigan. These three volumes have information on the collections and services of over 13,000 special collections, libraries, and information centers.

World Guide to Libraries. R. R. Bowker Co., N.Y. This 2-volume set will help you find material that is unavailable in American libraries. It lists over 40,000 public, university, and special libraries in over 150 countries. Specialty collections often offer information that is not available anywhere else.

American Library Directory. R. R. Bowker Co., N.Y. If you can't find what you want in a local library, this directory lists 25,000 American and 2,000 Canadian libraries.

Subject Collections (a guide to special book collections in libraries). R. R. Bowker Company, New York. This important research tool lists holdings in various libraries by subject as well as special collections.

American Booktrade Directory. R. R. Bowker Company, N.Y.. This directory contains the names and addresses of most of the publishers and booksellers in the country.

The New York Times Index—1851 to Date. Published by the New York Times. Newspaper articles are a good source of information. The Times articles are indexed by subject. In addition to providing access to articles from the premiere paper in the country, it will guide you to articles in your local paper as well.

University Microfilms, O.P. Books. Ann Arbor, Michigan. This organization compiled tens of thousands of out-of-print books on microfilm. For a fee, they will provide a printed copy of books on demand. This service is an excellent source for hard-to-find works.

University Microfilms. Ann Arbor, Michigan. Dissertations and theses are an important source of original research. Ask for their Datrix Ordering Information, a kit that enables you to order a printout on any topic. The printouts are arranged by key words. You may have to supply several key words in order to receive listings or appropriate material.

Research Centers Directory. Ann Arbor, Michigan. This directory consists of research information conducted by various colleges and universities.

Local College, University, Community College, and High School Libraries. In addition to many sources listed in this guide, these educational libraries are often staffed with scholars who have expertise in your field.

The National Union Catalog. Mansell, London. When this 610-volume work is completed, it will be the ultimate resource. In will list the holdings of the Library of Congress and catalog the holdings of the other major U.S. and Canadian libraries.

U.S. Superintendent of Documents. Washington, D.C. The U.S. Government publishes thousands of books, pamphlets, and articles on a wide range of topics each year. Consult your librarian or the Superintendent of Documents to determine which local libraries are repositories of government publications. Many libraries have cumulative listings of these publications.

Books for College Libraries. American Library Association, Chicago, Illinois This listing of 50,000 scholarly titles can help you find books that are not available in public libraries. This listing is useful because it is annotated.

The National Faculty Directory. Gale Research, Detroit, Michigan. Over 400,000 members of colleges, universities, and community colleges in the U.S. and Canada are listed. Many of them will probably be working in the area you are researching.

Union Lists of Serials in Libraries of the United States and Canada. H. H. Wilson Company, Bronx, New York. If you are looking for magazine articles, this directory lists over 150,000 serials found in nearly 1,000 libraries. It can help you to obtain photocopies of articles.

State Library. Your library can borrow from vast holdings of your state library. Most libraries maintain a union card file of the state holdings. Ask your librarian.

Inter-Library Loans. Most libraries participate in an inter-library loan system. If a book you want is not at a local library, you may be able to obtain it from another facility.

The Center for Research Libraries. Chicago, Illinois. This excellent research center holds millions of books and microfilms. Your local library, or one near you, may be a member. You may be able to borrow material.

Constance M. Winchell's Guide to Reference Books. American Library Association, Chicago, Illinois. This listing of over 8,000 reference books is the most important and comprehensive guide to reference books available.

Guide to Theses and Dissertations. Gale Research, Detroit, Michigan. This annotated, international bibliography of bibliographies will lead you to theses and dissertations from institutions of higher learning all over the world.

Ulrich's International Periodicals Directory. R. R. Bowker Co., N.Y. This directory, used primarily by scholars, lists publications arranged by subject.

The Bibliographia Index, March 1938 to Date. H. W. Wilson Company, Bronx, New York. This semi-annual index lists large book and small magazine bibliographies.

The Reader's Guide to Periodical Literature, 1900 to Date. H. W. Wilson Company, Bronx, New York. Articles that have been published from 1900 to the present in 160 popular magazines are indexed in this guide. Many libraries have computerized versions of this large set of books to make finding appropriate articles faster and easier.

Guides to Reprints. NCR/Microcard Editions, Washington, D.C. One problem with using older bibliographies is that many of the books are listed as out-of-print from their original publishers. This guide lists tens of thousands of books that have been reprinted and are now available.

The National Archives. Washington, D.C. The National Archives maintains permanent records of government documents. Write and ask about their specific holdings. You will receive a list of what they have in your general subject area.

Library of Congress. Washington, D.C. This is a source for millions of books, articles, and films in all subjects. To access holdings, check your key words against the subject headings in the Dictionary Catalog of the Library of Congress. They use a different numbering system than most local libraries. Get a reference number for your key word; use it to make inquiries for items. Order a book on microfilm, hard copy, or microcopy. Or subscribe to a monthly publication of titles in a particular classification number; receive catalog cards of new books.

Association of College and Research Libraries. American Library Association, Chicago, Illinois. This group helps you find college and research libraries in your field.

Special Libraries Association. Washington, D.C. Contact this organization for libraries with special collections on particular topics.

National Directory of Addresses and Telephone Numbers. General Information, Inc. A directory of 200,000 addresses and phone numbers for associations, corporations, and government agencies.

New York Times Index. The New York Times. You can use this index to locate information by checking under "key word" listings. Many libraries have this material on microfilm.

The Yellow Pages. The Yellow Pages for major cities can help you to find specialty book stores. Your library probably has sets of telephone books from around the country.

Information U.S.A. Information U.S.A., Chevy Chase, Maryland. Mathew Lesko is an expert at finding information sources within the U.S. Government. Read his company's monthly newsletter or his book, *Information U.S.A.* (Penguin).

Government Information & Resources

Consumer Information Catalog, Consumer Info. Center, P.O. Box 100, Pueblo, Colorado 81002. This catalog lists free and low-cost federal publications of consumer interest. Topics include: federal benefits, drugs, exercise, financial planning, health, hearing aids, hobbies, food, medical problems, mental health, nutrition, small business, sources of assistance, weight control, etc.

United States Government Information, U.S. Government Printing Office, Superintendent of Documents, Washington, D.C. 20402. Telephone: (202) 512-1800 (8 am to 4 pm Eastern time); Fax: (202) 512-2250 (anytime). Publications, periodicals, and electronic products/databases on: business, disabilities, education, environmental science, family, government references, health, etc.

U.S. Government Books, U.S. Government Printing Office, Superintendent of Documents, Washington, D.C. 20402. Telephone: (202) 783-3238 (8 am - 4 pm Eastern time); Fax: (202) 512-2250 (anytime). Publications for sale by the U.S. Government Printing Office. Call or write for a catalog.

U.S. Government Information For Business, U.S. Government Printing Office, Superintendent of Documents, Washington, D.C. 20402. Telephone: (202) 512-1526; Fax: (202) 512-1262.

National Self-Help & Holistic Health Numbers & Organizations

This list provides some national resources for information on healing and recovery. Check your telephone directory yellow pages under "Community Services" for local help or resources. Or get the AT&T Toll-Free 800 Directory, Consumer Edition. To order, call: 1 (800) 426-8686. This directory contains the 800 Consumer White Pages, an alphabetical listing by name of businesses, government agencies, and organizations with 800 numbers.

AIDS / HIV Hotline: (800) 342-AIDS (or 2437). TDD (hearing impaired) Hotline: (800) 243-7889. Spanish speaking: (800) 344-7432. For info., resources, referrals, and a national database for support services, treatment options, and test sites in your area. Open 24 hours/day, 7 days/week.

Alcoholics Anonymous (AA), General Service Office, 475 Riverside Dr., New York, N.Y. 10115. (212) 870-3400.

American Anorexia/Bulimia Association, Inc., 418 East 76th St., New York, N.Y. 10021. (212) 891-8686.

American Association of Naturopathic Physicians, 2366 Eastlake Ave., Suite 322, Seattle, Washington 98102. (206) 323-7610.

American Chronic Pain Association, P.O. Box 850, Rocklin, CA 95677. (916) 632-0922.

American Diabetes Association. (800) 232-3472.

The American Foundation of Traditional Chinese Medicine, 1280 Columbus Ave., Suite 302, San Francisco, CA 94133. (415) 776-0502.

The American Heart Association. (800) 242-8721.

The American Holistic Health Association, P.O. Box 17400, Anaheim, CA 92817. (714) 779-6152.

American Self-Help Clearinghouse, St. Clares-Riverside Medical Center, Denville, N.J. 07834. (201) 625-7101. (8:30 am - 5:00 pm Eastern time)

The Biofeedback & Psychophysiology Clinic, The Menniger Clinic, P.O. Box 829, Topeka, KS 66601-0829. (913) 273-7500.

Cancer Information Service. (800) 4-CANCER.

Chronic Fatigue Syndrome information line at the Centers for Disease Control. CDC maintains a 24-hour voice information system that provides up-to-date information on this illness. (404) 332-4555.

Eating Disorder Organization, 1925 East Dublin Granville Road, Columbus, OH 43229-3517. (614) 436-1112.

ECap (Exceptional Cancer Patients), 1302 Chapel St., New Haven, CT 06511. (203) 865-8392.

Human Ecology Action League, P.O. Box 49126, Atlanta, Georgia 30359. (404) 248-1898. Help/support for people with environmental illness.

Institute of Noetic Sciences, P.O. Box 909, Dept. M, Sausalito, CA 94966-0909. (800) 383-1394. Publications on medicine, spirituality, science.

The Mind-Body Medical Institute, 185 Pilgrim Road, Boston, MA 02215. (617) 732-7000.

National Council on Alcoholism and Drug Dependency (NCADD), 12 West 21st St., New York, N.Y., 10010. (212) 206-6770.

National Health Information Center, P.O. Box 1133, Washington, D.C. 20013-1133. (800) 336-4797.

National Self-Help Clearinghouse, 25 West 43rd St., Rm. 620, New York, N.Y. 10036. (212) 642-2944.

Overeaters Anonymous, National Office, 383 Van Ness Ave., Ste. 1601, Torrance, CA 90501. (310) 618-8835.

Project Inform, 1965 Market Street, Suite 220, San Francisco, CA 94103. (415) 558-8669. (AIDS / HIV information and newsletter)

The Stress Reduction Clinic, Dept. of Medicine, University of Massachusetts Medical Center, Worcester, MA 01655. (508) 856-1616.

World Research Foundation, 15300 Ventura Blvd., Suite 405, Sherman Oaks, CA 91403. (818) 907-5483. (Information on health issues.)

Recommended Self-Help & Healing Books, Products & Tapes

Bargain Books, Edward R. Hamilton Bookseller, Falls Village, CT 06031-5000. Save up to 80% on publihsers' overstocks, remainders, imports, reprints. America's biggest selection on bargain books. Thousands of titles. Order catalog.

Books On Tape, Inc. ®. Call: (800) 626-3333 for a free color brochure. World's largest selection of audio books. Best sellers on cassette; more than 3,000 current and classic favorites. Twenty new titles monthly. All full-length.

The Best Catalogs In The World, Publisher Inquiry Services, 951 Broken Sound Parkway NW, Bldg. 190, P.O. Box 5057, Boca Raton, FL 33431-0857.

John Bradshaw, P.O. Box 980547, Houston, TX 77098. (713) 529-9437.

CFIDS Buyers Club, 1187 Coast Village Road, #1-280, Santa Barbara, CA 93108. 1-800-366-6056. Fax: 1-805-565-3946. (Order their catalog of natural supplements and health resources.)

The Complete Guide To Exercise Videos™. For catalog: 1-800-433-6769.

Environmental Health Shopper™, P. O. Box 239, Fate, TX 75132. 1-800-447-1100. (Catalog of home-health care products to help reduce pollutants.)

Future Medicine Publishing. 10124-18th St. Court East, Puyallup, WA 98371. (800) 720-6363. (*Alternative Medicine: Definitive Guide*, *Alternative Medicine Yellow Pages*, *Natural Home Remedies*, or *Alternative Medicine Digest*.)

Marilyn Gordon/Wise Word Publishing, P.O. Box 10795, Oakland, CA 94610. (510) 839-4800 (self-hypnosis books and tapes).

John Gray, Ph.D. 20 Sunnyside Ave., Ste A-130, Mill Valley, CA 94941. (800) 821-3033 (seminars, books, tapes).

Hay House, 1154 E. Dominguez, Carson, CA 90746. (800) 654-5126.

Hunter House, P.O. Box 2914, Alameda, CA 94501-0914. To order a catalog of books on women's health and self-help/psychology, call: (800) 266-5592.

Impact Publishers, P.O. Box 1094, San Luis Obispo, CA 93406. (805) 543-5911; Fax (805) 543-4093. (Order a catalog of caregiving and self-help books.)

Gerald Jampolsky, M.D., c/o **Center for Attitudinal Healing**, 33 Buchanan Drive, Sausalito, CA 94965. (415) 331-6161.

The Mail Order Catalog, P.O. Box 180, Summertown, TN 38483. (800) 695-2241. (A catalog of vegetarian and alternative health books, and health foods.)

New Harbinger Self-Help Catalog, 5674 Shattuck Ave., Oakland, CA 94609. (800) 748-6273 (Order their catalog of health and self-help/psychology books.)

Publications International, 7373 N. Cicero Ave., Lincolnwood, IL 60646.

The Pyramid Collection™, P.O. Box 3333, Altid Park - Chelmsford, Mass. 01824-0933. (800) 333-4220 (Catalog of personal growth & exploration, includes: healing products, tapes, books, gifts, clothing, candles, crystals, etc.)

The Vitamin Trader, (800) 334-9310 (Healthy Discounts on Quality Vitamins.)

Whole Person Associates, 210 West Michigan, Duluth, MN 55802-1908. (800) 247-6789. (Order their catalog: "Stress & Wellness Resources for Trainers, Consultants, and Educators." It includes group exercises, relaxation tapes, and wellness video tapes.)

Chapter 14. References / Recommended Reading & Tapes

Business / Financial / Self-Employment Books

Arden, L. *The Work-At-Home Sourcebook*. Boulder, CO: Live Oak Publ., 1994. This book lists over 1,000 companies (by state) that routinely use qualified home workers. It provides specifics for each company, such as pay scale and work requirements.

Boldt, L. G. *Zen & The Art of Making a Living: A practical guide to creative career design*. New York: Penguin Books, 1993.

Brabec, B. *Homemade Money: The Definitive Guide to Success in a Home Business*. White Hall, Virginia: Betterway Publications, 1994. How to get started, select the right home business, avoid the wrong ones, and plan for profits and success. An A- Z course in business basics, including: selling direct and selling to wholesale markets; strategies for diversification and expansion; and 500 information-by-mail resources.

Dominquez, J., and V. Robin. *Your Money or Your Life: Transforming Your Relationship with Money & Achieving Financial Independence*. New York: Penguin, 1992.

Edwards, P. and S. Edwards. *Working From Home: Everything You Need To Know About Living and Working Under The Same Roof*. New York: Putnam, 1994.

———. *The Best Home Businesses For The '90s: The Inside Information You Need To Know To Select A Home-Based Business That's Right For You*. N.Y.: Putnam, 1991.

Ellsworth, J. H. and M. V. Ellsworth. *Using CompuServe: The Complete Guide to All the On-line Services and Resources Available*. Indianapolis, IN: D. P. Ewing, 1994.

Green, G. G. *How To Start & Manage Your Own Busines*. N.Y.: New Am. Library, 1987.

Hahn, H., and R. Stout. *The Internet Yellow Pages*. New York: McGraw Hill, 1994. A unique directory to find thousands of free Internet resources from around the world.

Hill, N. *Think & Grow Rich*. New York: Fawcett, 1960.

Holt, R. *How To Publish, Promote & Sell Your Own Book*. N.Y.: St. Martin's Press, 1985.

Kremer, J. *1001 Ways To Market Your Books*. Fairfield, Iowa: Ad-Lib Publ., 1990.

Levine, J.R., and C. Baroudi. *The Internet For Dummies*™. San Mateo, CA: IDG, 1993.

Mundis, J. *How To Get Out Of Debt, Stay Out Of Debt & Live Prosperously: Based on the Proven Principles & Techniques of Debtors Anonymous*. New York: Bantam, 1988.

Phillips, C. *The New Money Workbook for Women*. Andover, MA: Brick House, 1988.

Sinetar, M. *Do What You Love, The Money Will Follow: Discovering Your Right Livelihood*. New York: Paulist Press, 1987.

- Social Security Disability Benefits Information

Ross, J. W. *Social Security Disability Benefits: How To Get Them! How To Keep Them! A Guide For The Truly Disabled For The Fight Of Their Lives*. Slippery Rock, PA: Ross Publishing, 1984.

Smith, D. M. (Attorney at Law). *Disability Workbook For Social Security Applicants*. Order from: The CFIDS Association, P.O. Box 220398, Charlotte, NC 28222-0398.

Business / Financial / Self-Employment Catalogs

Entrepreneur Magazine Group's Small Business Development Catalog. Entrepreneur Magazine Group, 2392 Morse Avenue, P.O. Box 57050, Irvine, CA 92619-7050. Telephone: 1-800-421-2300. Fax: 1-714-851-9088. A catalog of over 200 start-up guides, books, and software to help you succeed in a business of your own.

Mailing List Catalog. Telephone: 1-800-966-LIST. A catalog with mailing lists of over 80 million consumer households and over 9 million business addresses.

Caregiving Books

Jarrett, R. M. *Caring For The Caregiver: A Nurse's Journey to Health and Inner Peace* . Beaverton, Oregon: Happy Talk Books, 1993. The author offers honest and insightful caregiving tips on keeping mentally, physically, and emotionally fit while taking care of others. She includes a wealth of reference materials.

Lowe, P. C. *Care Pooling: How to Get the Help You Need to Care for the Ones You Love*. San Francisco: Berrett-Koehler Publishers, 1993. The author offers ways for caregivers to get more help and support. Tools are provided for: identifying potential carepoolers (a network of support), understanding why it is hard to ask for help, initiating carepooling relationships, creating written guidelines, resolving conflicts among carepoolers, and hiring a shared care provider.

Pohl, M., and D. J. Kay. *Staying Sane: When You Care For Someone With Chronic Illness: Creative Ideas And Activities To Brighten Your Day*. Deerfield Beach, FL: Health Communications, 1993. Creative ideas and activities to brighten your day and to keep your spirits up. Ways to care for loved ones, while taking care of your own needs. An upbeat, motivational book to lighten the heavy burden of caregiving. It shows ways to care for others without losing yourself. If you're a wife, husband, family member, nurse, counselor, friend, or lover of someone who is chronically ill, you need support.

Chronic Fatigue Syndrome Audio Tapes

Berne, K. Chronic Fatigue Syndrome (information, relaxation, and healing exercises); CFS: For Those Who Care; CFS & Self-Esteem; Neurocognitive Aspects of CFS. Write: BHB Communications, 761 E. University, Suite F, Mesa, AZ 85203.

Collinge, W. <u>Recovering From CFS: The Home Self-Empowerment Program</u>. Tapes cover healing imagery, deep relaxation, breathing exercises, sleep enhancement, and mind/body medicine. To order, call Dr. William Collinge: 1 (800) 745-1837.

Chronic Fatigue Syndrome Booklet

"The Facts About Chronic Fatigue Syndrome" (August 1994). U.S. Department of Health and Human Services, Public Health Service, Centers for Disease Control and Prevention. Atlanta, Georgia 30333.

Chronic Fatigue Syndrome Books

Bell, D. S. *The Doctor's Guide to Chronic Fatigue Syndrome.* Addison-Wesley, 1994.

———. *Chronic Fatigue Immune Dysfunction Syndrome: The Disease of a Thousand Names.* New York: Pollard Publications, 1991. Write: Pollard Publications, P.O. Box 180, Lyndonville, N.Y. 14098. Call: (716) 765-2060.

Berne, K. *CFIDS Lite: Chronic Fatigue Immune Dysfunction Syndrome with One-Third the Seriousness.* Mesa, AZ: BHB Communications, 1991.

———. *Running On Empty: CFIDS.* Hunter House, 1992.

Brooks, B. and N. Smith. *CFIDS: An "Owner's Manual."* BBNS Publishers, Box 6456, Silver Spring, MD 20916-6456.

Collinge, W. *Recovering From Chronic Fatigue Syndrome: A Guide To Self-Empowerment.* New York: Putnam, 1993.

Feiden, K. *Hope and Help for C.F.S.* New York: Prentice Hall, 1992.

Fisher, G.C. *Chronic Fatigue Syndrome: A Victim's Guide To Understanding, Treating & Coping With This Debilitating Disease.* New York: Warner Books, 1989.

Goldstein, J. *Chronic Fatigue Syndrome: The Struggle for Health: A Diagnostic and Treatment Guide for Patients and Their Physicians.* Beverly Hills, CA: CFS Institute, 1990. Write: CFS Institute, 436 N. Roxbury Drive, Suite 110, Beverly Hills, CA 90210.

Hale, M., and C. Miller. *The Chronic Fatigue Syndrome Cookbook.* Carol, 1994.

Jacobs, P. D. *Chronic Fatigue Syndrome: How To Find Facts And Get Help.* San Francisco, CA: PDJ Publishing, 1995. Write: PDJ, 750 La Playa, #647, San Francisco, CA 94121.

Lewis, K. S. *Successful Living With A Chronic Illness.* Wayne, NJ: Avery, 1985.

Pitzele, Zefra. *We Are Not Alone: Learning To Live With A Chronic Illness.* New York: Workman Publishing, 1985.

Rosenbaum, M., and M. Susser. *Solving the Puzzle of Chronic Fatigue Syndrome.* Tacoma, WA: Life Sciences Press, 1992. Life Sciences Press, P.O. Box 1174, Tacoma, WA 98401.

Solomon, N. *Sick & Tired of Being Sick & Tired.* N.Y.: Wynwood Press, 1989.

Stoff, J. A., and C. Pellegrino. *CFS: The Hidden Epidemic.* N.Y.: Random House, 1988.

Chronic Fatigue Syndrome Journals

The CFIDS Chronicle: Journal of the Chronic Fatigue & Immune Dysfunction Syndrome Association. Write: The CFIDS Association, Inc., Community Health Services, P.O. Box 220398, Charlotte, NC 28222-0398. (704) 362-2343; FAX: (704) 365-9755.

Diagnosis & Treatment. The Chronic Fatigue Syndrome: A Comprehensive Approach to Its Definition and Study. U. S. Dept. of Health & Human Services. Public Health Service. CDC, Mailstop A-15, Atlanta, Georgia 30333.

Chronic Fatigue Syndrome Information Line

Call: (900) 896-2343 ($2 for the first minute; $1 each additional minute.)

Chronic Fatigue Syndrome/ME Computer Network
Chronic Fatigue Syndrome/ME (myalgic encephalomyelitis) Networking Project, P. O. Box 1147, Washington, D.C. 20008. Send a self-addressed, stamped legal-size envelope with a donation for a brochure on electronic networking information.

Chronic Fatigue Syndrome Video Tapes
The following tapes are available through the CFIDS Association of America. Call: (704) 365-9755 or write: The CFIDS Assoc., P.O. Box 220398, Charlotte, NC 28222.

"CFS Diagnosis & Treatment: A Grand Rounds Medical Training Video." 30 min., $30. Kaiser Permanente, 1995. Jonathan Rest, M.D. instructs healthcare professionals on the diagnosis and treatment of CFIDS. Based on the 1994 CFS case definition.
"Living Hell: The Real World of Chronic Fatigue Syndrome." 1 hour tape, $32. Directed by Lenny Copeland of Authentic Productions, 1993.
"Patient-Oriented Conference." 4-1/2 hrs, $35. The CFIDS Association of America, 1995.
"CFIDS Support Network Meeting." 2 hrs, $12. The CFIDS Association of America, '95.

Chronic Illness Audio Tapes
"Relaxation, Imagery, and Healing Exercises" by Katrina H. Berne, Ph.D. BHB Communications, 1996. 1 hour tape, $9. Daytime and evening exercises to reduce tension and promote healing. Call The CFIDS Association of America: (704) 365-9755.
Self-healing tape programs for cancer, chronic fatigue syndrome, fibromyalgia, HIV, heart disease, hypertension, gastrointestinal disorders, preparation for surgery, stress reduction, and health enhancement. Call Dr. William Collinge: (800) 745-1837.

Chronic Illness Books

Duff, Kat. *The Alchemy of Illness: A woman explores the transforming—and paradoxically, healing—experience of being ill*. New York: Pantheon Books, 1993.

Hanner, L. and J. J. Witek. *When You're Sick and Don't Know Why: Coping With Your Undiagnosed Illness*. Minneapolis, MN: DCI Publishing, 1991.

Lorig, K., H. Holman, D. Sobel, D. Laurent, V. Gonzalez, and M. Minor. *Living a Healthy Life with Chronic Conditions*. Palo Alto, CA: Bull Publishing, 1994.

Pollin, I., and S. K. Golant. *Taking Charge: Overcoming the Challenges of Long-Term Illness*. New York: Times Books, 1994.

Communication Books

Elgin, S. H. *The Gentle Art of Verbal Self Defense*. N.Y.: Prentice-Hall, 1980.

———. *More on the Gentle Art of Verbal Self-Defense*. N.Y.: Prentice-Hall, Inc., 1983.

Evans, P. *The Verbally Abusive Relationship: How to Recognize It and How to Respond*. Holbrook MA: Bob Adams, Publishers, 1992.

Ray, S. *Loving Relationships. The Secrets of a Great Relationship*. Berkeley, CA: Celestial Arts, 1992.

Smith, M. J. *When I Say No, I Feel Guilty: How to Cope–Using the Skills of Systematic Assertive Therapy*. New York: Bantam Books, 1975.

Tannen, D. *You Just Don't Understand*. New York: Ballantine Books, 1990.

Disabilities Resources

The Alliance for Technology Access. *Computer Resources For People With Disabilities: A Guide To Exploring Today's Assistive Technology*. Alameda, CA: Hunter House, 1994.

This book shows how America's 45 million people with disabilities can use computer technology to achieve goals and change their lives. It helps readers to define their needs, develop a technology plan, build a supportive team, and make decisions. It explains the ADA, IDEA, Tech Act, and other legislation. Readers learn how to identify appropriate computer technology, seek funding to purchase it, set it up, and use it at work, school, or home. It lists support groups, agencies, professional associations, and educational training institutions that offer many options to people with disabilities. The Alliance for Technology Access is a network of community-based technology resource centers, dedicated to providing information, resources, and support to people with disabilities and increasing their access to standard and assistive technologies.

San Mateo County Commission on Disabilities. "Emergency Preparedness for People With Special Needs" (booklet). Write: 225 West 37th Avenue, San Mateo, CA 94403.

Environmental Booklets & Catalogs

Consumer Information Center, P.O. Box 100, Pueblo, CO 81002. Write for booklets on environmental information, including: "Home Buyer's Guide to Environmental Hazards" (a 41-page booklet which covers lead and other environmental risks and what to do about them); and "Getting the Lead Out" (a 6-page FDA booklet).

The Natural Bedroom: All natural bedding. Call for a catalog: (800) 365-6563.

The Natural House Catalog: Everything You Need To Create an Environmentally Friendly Home by David Pearson. A Fireside Book, published by Simon & Schuster, 1996.

The Cotton Place – Your Connection to Good Things from Nature's Fibers, P.O. Box 59721, Dallas, TX 75229. For information, call: (800) 451-8866.

Environmental Health Books

Breecher, M. M., and S. Linde. *Healthy Homes in a Toxic World: Preventing, Identifying, & Eliminating Hidden Health Hazards in Your Home*. New York: J. Wiley, 1992.

Center for Study of Responsive Law. *The Home Book: A Guide to Safety, Security and Savings in the Home*. Introduction by Ralph Nader. Washington, D.C., 1991. Write: *The Home Book*, P.O. Box 19367, Washington, D.C. 20036.

Dadd, D. L. *The Nontoxic Home & Office: Protecting Yourself and Your Family from Everyday Toxics and Health Hazards. Eliminate Indoor Pollution & Sick Building Syndrome*. New York: St. Martin's Press, 1992.

EarthWorks Group. *50 Simple Things You Can Do To Save The Earth*. Berkeley, CA: EarthWorks Press, 1989. Write: EarthWorks Press, Box 25, 1400 Shattuck Ave., Berkeley, CA 94709. Or call: 510-527-5811.

Ehrlich, P. R., and A. H. Ehrlich. *The Population Explosion: The Indispensable Guide To Understanding & Solving Today's #1 Environmental Problem*. New York: A Touchstone, Simon & Schuster, 1990.

Hunter, L. M. *The Healthy Home: An Attic-To-Basement Guide To Toxin-Free Living*. New York: Pocket Books, 1990.

Kibbey, D. *Building Naturally: A Guide to Professionals and a Compendium of Articles*. 1994. Natural Building Network, P.O. Box 1110, Sebastopol, CA 95473.

Lappé, M. *Chemical Deception*. Sierra Publishing, 1991.

MacEachern, D. *Save Our Planet: 750 Everyday Ways You Can Help Clean Up The Earth*. New York: Dell Publishing, 1990.

Null, G. *Clearer, Cleaner, Safer, Greener: A Blueprint For Detoxifying Your Environment*. New York: Villard Books, 1990.

Rogers, S A. *The E.I. Syndrome: An Rx for Environmental Illness. Are You Allergic To The 21st Century?* New York: Prestige Publishers, 1986. Write: Prestige Publ., Box 3161, 3502 Brewerton Road, Syracuse, NY 13220.

Rousseau, D., W. J. Rea, and J. Enwright. *Your Home, Your Health, and Well-Being: What You Can Do To Design Or Renovate Your House Or Apartment To Be Free of Outdoor And Indoor Pollution.* Vancouver, B.C.: Hartley & Marks, Ltd., 1989. Write: Hartley & Marks, Ltd., 3663 West Broadway, Vancouver, B.C., V6R 2B8.

Venolia, C. *Healing Environments: Your Guide To Indoor Well-Being.* Berkeley: Celestial Arts, 1988.

Environmental Newsletters

The New Reactor, c/o Environmental Health Network — P.O. Box 1155, Larkspur, CA 94977. Voice Mail: (415) 541-5075.

Healthy Home & Workplace, 248 Lafayette Street, New York, N.Y. 10012

Exercise Books

Bailey, C. *Smart Exercise: Burning Fat, Getting Fit.* New York: Houghton Mifflin, 1994.

Bell, L., and E. Seyfer. *Gentle Yoga: A Guide to Gentle Exercise.* Berkeley, CA: Celestial Arts, 1982. Yoga for people with illness (arthritis, M.S., stroke damage) or disabilities.

Cooper, R. K. *Health & Fitness Excellence.* Boston: Houghton Mifflin, 1989.

Eastman, R., with P. Ryan. *Full Circle Fitness: Be Your Own Personal Trainer.* New York: William Morrow, 1990.

Gordon, N. F. *Chronic Fatigue: Your Complete Exercise Guide. The Cooper Clinic & Research Institute Fitness Series.* Champaign, IL: Human Kinetics Publishers, 1993.

Park Nicollet Medical Foundation. *Over 50 & Fit: A program to enhance flexibility, strength and stamina.* Minneapolis, MN: CompCare Publishers, 1991.

Rippe, J. M. *Fit For Success.* New York: Prentice Hall Press, 1989.

Health & Science Journals, Magazines & Newsletters

Alternative Medicine Digest, a bi-monthly journal. Call: 1-800-720-6363.

Delicious! Your Magazine of Natural Living. Published monthly by New Hope Communications Inc., 1301 Spruce St., Boulder, CO 80302. (303) 939-8440.

Nutrition and Your Health. New Health Network, 1301 Spruce St. Boulder, CO 80302. (800) 933-8440.

Mental Medicine Update, The Center for Health Sciences, P.O. Box 381062, Cambridge, MA 02238-1062. (800) 222-4745. (The Mind/Body Health Newsletter.)

Science News, 1719 North West St., Wash. D.C. 20036. Call: 1-800-247-2160.

The Wellness Letter by the School of Public Health at the University of California at Berkeley. This monthly, 8-page newsletter has useful information on health, nutrition, exercise, and prevention of illness. Write to: P. O. Box 420148, Palm Coast, FL 32142.

Spectrum®: The Wholistic News Magazine. (ISSN 1049-9075) 6 times a year by the Spectrum Universal Corp., 61 Dutile Rd., Belmont, NH 03220-5252. (603) 528-4710.

Holistic Health Books

Adamson, E. *Art As Healing.* Boston: Coventure, Ltd., 1990.

Atkinson, H. *Women and Fatigue: Life-Changing Help For Your Personal Energy Crisis!* New York: Pocket Books, 1987.

Benson, H. and E. M. Stuart. *The Wellness Book: The Comprehensive Guide to Maintaining Health and Treating Stress-Related Illness*. N.Y.: Simon & Schuster, 1992.

Berger, S. M. *What Your Doctor Didn't Learn In Medical School*. N.Y.: Avon Books, 1989.

Berkeley Holistic Health Center. *The Holistic Health Handbook: A Tool for Attaining Wholeness of Body, Mind, and Spirit*. Berkeley: And/Or Press.

Birkedahl, N. *Older & Wiser: A Workbook For Coping With Aging*. Oakland, CA: New Harbinger Publications, 1991. How to stay active; make decisions about money, insurance, wills; modify your diet; find the right exercise; adapt to limitations; deal with doctors; make the most of your personal resources; understand your changing feelings; and deal with the challenges of illness.

Bonk, M., ed. *Alternative Medicine Yellow Pages: The comprehensive guide to the new world of health*. Puyallup, Washington: Future Medicine Publishing, 1994.

Boyle, W., and A. Saine. *Lectures in Naturopathic Hydrotherapy*. East Palestine, OH: Buckeye Naturopathic Press, 1988.

Borysenko, J., with L. Rothstein. *Minding The Body, Mending The Mind*. New York: Bantam Books, 1988.

Brennan, B. A. *Light Emerging: The Journey Of Personal Healing*. N.Y.: Bantam, 1993.

——. *Hands of Light: A Guide to Healing Through The Human Energy Field*. New York: Bantam Books, 1988.

The Burton Goldberg Group. *Alternative Medicine: The Definitive Guide*. Puyallup, Washington: Future Medicine Publishing, 1993.

Carlson, R., and B. Shield, ed. *Healers on Healing*. Los Angeles: J. P. Tarcher, 1989.

Carter, M. *Body Reflexology: Healing at Your Fingertips*. New York: Parker, 1983.

Chaitow, L. *The Body / Mind Purification Program*. New York: Simon & Schuster, 1990.

Chia, M. *Awaken Healing Energy Through The Tao*. Santa Fe, N.M.: Aurora Press, 1983.

——. *Chi Self-Massage: The Taoist Way of Rejuvenation*. Huntington, New York: Healing Tao Books, 1986.

Chopra, D. *Perfect Health: The Complete Mind / Body Guide*. New York: Harmony, 1991.

Cichoke, A.J. *Enzymes & Enzyme Therapy*. New Canaan, CT: Keats Publishing, 1994.

Cooper, R. K. *Health & Fitness Excellence: The Scientific Action Plan*. Boston: Houghton Mifflin Company, 1989.

Cousins, N. *Anatomy of An Illness*. New York: Norton, 1979.

Crisp, T. *Dream Dictionary: An A to Z Guide to Understanding Your Unconscious Mind*. New York: Wing Books, 1990.

Crook, W. G. *Detecting Your Hidden Allergies*. Jackson, TN: Professional Books, 1988.

Dossey, L. *Meaning & Medicine: Lessons from a Doctor's Tales of Breakthrough and Healing*. New York: Bantam Books, 1991.

Editors of *Prevention* ® Magazine. *Your Emotional Health and Well-Being*. Stamford, CT: Longmeadow Press, 1989.

Gach, M. R. *Greater Energy At Your Fingertips: How To Easily Increase Your Vitality In Ten Minutes*. Berkeley: Celestial Arts, 1986.

Gawain, S. *Living in the Light: A Guide to Personal and Planetary Transformation*. San Rafael, CA: New World Library, 1986.

Gray, J. *What You Feel You Can Heal*. Mill Valley, CA: Heart Publ., 1994.

Hay, L. L. *The Power Is Within You*. Carson, CA: Hay House, Inc., 1991.

Horvilleur, A. *The Family Guide To Homeopathy*. Virginia: Health & Homeopathy, 1986.

Jackson, R. *Massage Therapy: The holistic way to physical and mental health*. New York: Sterling Publishing, 1989.

Jarmey, C.; J. Tindall. *Acupressure for Common Ailments*. N.Y.: Simon & Schuster, 1991.

Justice, B. *Who Gets Sick: How Beliefs, Moods, and Thoughts Affect Your Health*. Los Angeles, CA: Jeremy P. Tarcher, 1988.

Lange, M. *Basically Balanced: A Wellness Guide for the Body, Mind, Heart, and Soul*. Chicago, IL: Sourcebooks Trade, 1994.

Lark, S. M. *Anxiety & Stress: A Self-Help Program*. Los Altos, CA: Westchester, 1993.

Levine, S. *Healing into Life and Death*. New York: Doubleday, 1987.

Liberman, J. *Light: Medicine of the Future*. Santa Fe, N.M.: Bear & Co. Publ., 1993.

Lidell, L., with S. Thomas, C. B. Cooke, and A. Porter. *The Book of Massage: The Complete Step-by-Step Guide to Eastern and Western Techniques*. N.Y.: Simon & Schuster, 1984.

Melville, A., and C. Johnson. *Health Without Drugs: Alternatives to Prescription and Over-the-Counter Medicines. Including Diet, Exercise And Stress Reduction*. New York: Simon & Schuster, 1991.

Mendelsohn, R. S. *Confessions of a Medical Heretic*. Chicago: Warner, 1979.

Miller, E. E., with D. Lueth. *Self Imagery: Creating Your Own Good Health*. Berkeley: Celestial Arts, 1978.

Null, G. *Healing Your Body Naturally: Alternative treatments...* N.Y.: Wings Books, 1992.

Ohashi, W., V. Lindner, ed. *Do It Yourself Shiatsu: How To Perform The Ancient Japanese Art Of Acupuncture Without Needles*. New York: E.P. Dutton, 1976.

Ornstein, R., and D. Sobel. *Healthy Pleasures*. Menlo Park, CA: Addison-Wesley, 1989.

Pinckney, C. *Callanetics: 10 Years Younger In 10 Hours*. New York: Avon Books, 1984.

Ponder, C. *The Dynamic Laws Of Healing*. Marina del Rey, CA: DeVorss & Co., 1985.

Roman, S. *Living with Joy: Keys To Personal Power & Spiritual Transformation*. Tiburon, CA: H.J. Kramer, 1986.

Rossbach, S., and L. Yun. *Living Color: Master Lin Yun's Guide To Feng Shui And The Art Of Color*. New York: Kodansha America, 1994.

Ryan, R. S., and J. W. Travis. *Wellness Workbook*. Berkeley: Ten Speed Press, 1981.

Scalzo, R. *The Naturopathic Handbook of Herbal Formulas: A Practical & Concise Herb User's Guide*. Durango, CO: Kivaki Press, 1994.

Siegel, A. B. *Dreams That Can Change Your Life: Navigating Life's Passages Through Turning Point Dreams*. New York: Berkley Books, 1990.

Siegel, B. S. *Love, Medicine and Miracles*. New York: Harper & Row, 1986.

———. *Peace, Love and Healing*. New York: Harper & Row, 1989.

Sinetar, M. *Elegant Choices, Healing Choices: Finding Grace and Wholeness in Everything We Choose*. New York: Paulist Press, 1988.

Smith Jones, S. *Choose To Be Healthy: Discover How To Embrace Life And Live Fully*. Berkeley: Celestial Arts, 1987.

UCLA School of Public Health. *50 Simple Things You Can Do To Save Your Life*. Berkeley, CA: EarthWorks Press, 1992. Write: EarthWorks Press, 1400 Shattuck Avenue, #25, Berkeley, CA 94709.

Ullman, D. *Discovering Homeopathy: Medicine for the 21st Century. Your Introduction to the Science & Art of Homeopathic Medicine*. Berkeley, CA: No. Atlantic Books, 1991.

Unity. *Daily Word*. Unity Village, MO 64065.

Weil, A. *Natural Health, Natural Medicine: A Comprehensive Manual For Wellness And Self-Care*. Boston: Houghton Mifflin Company, 1990.

Wilson, M. B. *Thorsons Introductory Guide to Chiropractic*. London: HarperCollins, 1991.

Humor Books

Barry, D. *Stay Fit & Healthy*. Emmaus, Pennsylvania: Rodale Press, 1985.

Becker, S. *All I Need To Know I Learned From My Cat*. New York: Workman, 1990.

Eales, S. *Earthtoons: The First Book of Eco-Humor*. New York: Warner Books, 1971.

Josefsberg, M. *Comedy Writing For Television & Hollywood. A Book To Be Read For Fun...And Possibly For Profit*. New York: Harper & Row, 1987.

Klein, A. *The Healing Power Of Humor*. Los Angeles: J.P. Tarcher, 1989.

Kushner, M. *The Light Touch: How To Use Humor For Business Success*. New York: Simon & Schuster, 1990.

Orben, R. *2100 Laughs For All Occasions*. New York: Doubleday, 1983.

Humor Magazines

Journal of Nursing, Jocularity. (The Humor Magazine for Nurses.) P.O. Box 40416, Mesa, AZ 85274. Phone: (602) 835-6165. Fax: (602) 835-6922.

The Comedy Magazine. 5290 Overpass Road, Santa Barbara, CA 93111-2048. Phone for Editing & Circulation: (805) 964-7841. Fax: (805) 964-1073.

Meditation / Mindfulness Books

Denniston, D. *The Transcendental Meditation™ Book: How to Enjoy the Rest of Your Life*. Fairfield, Iowa: Fairfield Press, 1986.

Kabat-Zinn, J. *Full Catastrophe Living: Using the Wisdom of Your Body and Mind to Face Stress, Pain, and Illness*. The Program of the Stress Reduction Clinic at the University of Massachusetts Medical Center. New York, Dell Publishing, 1990.

Kabat-Zinn, J. *Wherever You Go, There You Are: Mindfulness Meditation in Everyday Life*. New York: Hyperion, 1994.

Kornfield, J. *A Path with Heart: A Guide Through the Perils and Promises of Spiritual Life*. New York: Bantam Books, 1993.

Nutrition, Herbs & Supplements Books

Appleton, N. *Lick the Sugar Habit*. New York: Avery Publishing, 1988.

Berger, S. M. *How To Be Your Own Nutritionist: Write Your Own Prescription For Vital Health & Energy!* New York: Avon Books, 1987.

Carper, J. *The Food Pharmacy: Dramatic New Evidence That Food Is Your Best Medicine*. New York: Bantam Books, 1989.

Crook, W. G. *The Yeast Connection: A Medical Breakthrough*. New York: Vintage, 1986.
———. *CFS & The Yeast Connection*. Jackson, TN: Professional Books, 1992.

Crook, W. G., and M. Hurt Jones. *The Yeast Connection Cookbook. A Guide to Good Nutrition & Better Health*. Jackson, TN: Professional Books, 1989.

Dunne, L. J. *Nutrition Almanac. Third Edition*. N.Y.: McGraw-Hill Publishing, 1990.

Haas, R. *Eat Smart, Think Smart: How To Use Nutrients and Supplements To Achieve Maximum Mental And Physical Performance*. New York: HarperCollins, 1994.

Hamilton, E. Nunnelley, E. N. Whitney, and F. Sienkiewicz Sizer. *Nutrition Concepts & Controversies*. Fifth Ed. St. Paul, MN: West Publishing, 1991.

Hamilton, G. *The Organic Garden Book*. New York: Dorling Kindersley, 1993.

Howell, E. *Enzyme Nutrition*. Wayne, N.J.: Avery Publishing Group, 1985.

Lapchick, J.M. *The Label Reader's Pocket Dictionary of Food Additives*. Minneapolis, MN: Chronimed Publishing, 1993.

McDougall, J. A. *The McDougall Program: 12 Days To Dynamic Health. The Revolutionary Health & Diet Program*. New York: Penguin Books, 1990.

Manahan, W. *Eat For Health: A Do-It-Yourself Guide for Solving Common Medical Problems*. Tiburon, CA: H.J. Kramer, 1988.

Mindell, E. *Vitamin Bible: The Definitive Book...* New York: Warner Books, 1985.

Pelton, R., and T. Pelton. *Mind Food & Smart Pills: A Sourcebook for the Vitamins, Herbs, & Drugs That Can Increase Intelligence, Improve Memory, & Prevent Brain Aging*. New York: Doubleday, 1989.

Schwartz, G. R. *In Bad Taste: The MSG Syndrome*. N.Y.: A Signet Book, 1990.

Tierra, M. *The Way of Herbs*. New York: Pocket Books, 1990.

Turner, K. *Self-Healing Cookbook: A Macrobiotic Primer For Healing Body, Mind, & Moods With Whole, Natural Foods*. Earthtones, Box 411, Vashon Island, WA 98070.

Weiner, M. A. *Earth Medicine, Earth Food: The Classic Guide To The Herbal Remedies & Wild Plants Of The North American Indians*. New York: Fawcett, 1980.

Winter, R. *A Consumer's Dictionary of Food Additives*. New York: Crown Trade, 1994.

Physical Health Books

Bevan, J. *Anatomy & Physiology*. New York: Simon & Schuster, 1978.

Chopra, D. *Quantum Healing: Exploring The Frontiers Of Body, Mind, Medicine*. New York: Bantam Books, 1990.

Cooper, P. J., ed. Better Homes and Gardens: *Woman's Health & Medical Guide*. Des Moines, Iowa: Meredith Corporation, 1981.

Creighton, B., D. Smith, and L. Young. *Understanding Laboratory Values*. Medical Resources, P.O. Box 1900, Paradise, CA 95967. (916) 872-8400.

Davidson, P. *Chronic Muscle Pain Syndrome*. New York: Berkley Books, 1989. Explores the cause of pain and fatigue. A 7-step method to offer some relief. The book addresses: muscle aches, pains, stiffness, fatigue, exhaustion, joint swelling, tension, and headaches. The author has practiced internal medicine and rheumatology for 25 years.

Editors of Prevention Magazine Health Books. *The Doctors Book of Home Remedies: Thousands of Tips and Techniques Anyone Can Use to Heal Everyday Health Problems*. New York: Bantam Books, 1991.

Glisan, B., with S. Hochschuler, the Editors of Consumer Guide, in association with the Texas Back Institute. *50 Ways To Ease Back Pain*. Lincolnwood, IL: Publ. Int'l, 1994.

Inlander, C. B., and The Staff of the People's Medical Society. *150 Ways to be a Savvy Medical Consumer*. New York: Wings Books, 1992.

——, and E. I. Pavalon. *Your Medical Rights: How to Become an Empowered Consumer*. Boston: Little, Brown & Co., 1990. Details a patient's medical rights. Helps you take charge of when, where, and how you will receive medical treatment and from whom.

——, and Ed Weiner. *Take This Book To The Hospital With You: A Consumer's Guide To Surviving Your Hospital Stay*. New York: Wings Books, 1991.

Ivker, R.S. *Sinus Survival: A Self-Help Guide for Allergies, Bronchitis, Colds, and Sinusitis*. New York: Putnam, 1992.

Joklik, W. K. *Virology. Third Edition*. East Norwalk, Connecticut: Appleton-Century-Crofts. 1988. Write: Appleton & Lange, 25 Van Zant St., E. Norwalk, CT 06855.

Mandell, M. and L. Scanlon. *Dr. Mandell's 5-Day Allergy Relief System*. New York: Harper & Row, 1988.

Ornish, D. *Program For Reversing Heart Disease: The Only System Scientifically Proven to Reverse Heart Disease Without Drugs or Surgery*. New York: Ballantine Books, 1990.

People's Medical Society. *Dial 800 for Health. Free Hotlines / Services*. N.Y.: Wings, 1993.

Rosenfeld, I. *The Best Treatment*. New York: Simon & Schuster, 1991.

Siegel, B. S. *Love, Medicine & Miracles*. New York: HarperCollins, 1988.

Psychology / Self-Help Books

Bay Area Self-Help Center. *Bay Area 12-Step Directory*. San Francisco: Bay Area Self-Help Center, 1992. Write: Bay Area Self-Help Center, 2398 Pine Street, San Francisco, CA 94115. Phone: (415) 921-4044 for support group information.

Bloomfield, M.D., Harold H. and Peter McWilliams. *How To Heal Depression*. Los Angeles, CA: Prelude Press, 1994. To order, call: 1-800-LIFE-101.

Bradshaw, J. *Homecoming: Reclaiming and Championing Your Inner Child*. New York: Bantam Books, 1990.

Brown, L. J. *Self-Actuated Healing*. Happy Camp, CA: Naturegraph Publishers, 1988.

Burns, D. *The Feeling Good Handbook*. New York: Penguin, 1989.

———. *Feeling Good: The New Mood Therapy*. New York: Penguin, 1980.

Chopich, E. J., and M. Paul. *Healing Your Aloneness: Finding Love & Wholeness Through Your Inner Child*. S.F.: Harper, 1990.

Copeland, M. E., with M. McKay. *The Depression Workbook: A Guide For Living With Depression And Manic Depression*. Oakland, CA: New Harbinger Publications, 1992.

Davis, M., E. R. Eshelman, and M. McKay. *The Relaxation & Stress Reduction Workbook*. Oakland, CA: New Harbinger Publications, 1995.

Dinkmeyer, D., and L. E. Losoncy. *The Encouragement Book: Becoming A Positive Person*. New York: Prentice Hall Press, 1980.

Foster, C. *The Family Patterns Workbook: Breaking Free From Your Past & Creating A Life Of Your Own*. New York: Perigee Books, 1993.

Gawain, S. *Creative Visualization*. New York: Bantam Books, 1982.

Hay, L. L. *Heart Thoughts: A Treasury Of Inner Wisdom*. Carson, CA: Hay House, 1990.

Helmstetter, S. *Choices: Discover Your 100 Most Important Life Choices. Manage Your Choices And You Will Manage Your Life!* New York: Pocket Books, 1989.

————. *Finding The Fountain Of Youth Inside Yourself: You Can Grow Younger Every Day*. New York: Pocket Books, 1990.

————. *What To Say When You Talk To Your Self: Powerful New Techniques to Program Your Potential for Success*. New York: Pocket Books, 1982.

————. *The Self-Talk Solution: Take Control of Your Life—With the Self Management Program for Success!* New York: Pocket Books, 1987.

Jampolsky, G. *Out of Darkness, Into The Light: Inner Healing*. New York: Bantam, 1989.

Keyes, K. *The Power Of Unconditional Love: 21 Guidelines For Beginning, Improving, And Changing Your Most Meaningful Relationships*. Coos Bay, OR: Love Line, 1990.

Kushner, H.S. *When Bad Things Happen To Good People*. N.Y.: Schocken Books, 1981.

Lakein, A. *How To Get Control Of Your Time And Your Life*. N.Y.: A Signet Book, 1973.

McGrath, E. *When Feeling Bad is Good: An innovative self-help program for women to convert "healthy" depression into new sources of growth & power*. N.Y.: Bantam, 1992.

McKay, M., and P. Fanning. *Self-Esteem: A Proven Program Of Cognitive Techniques For Assessing, Improving, And Maintaining Your Self-Esteem*. Oakland, CA: New Harbinger Publications, 5674 Shattuck Ave., Oakland, CA 94609. Second ed., 1992.

————, P. D. Rogers, and J. McKay. *When Anger Hurts: Quieting The Storm Within*. Oakland, CA: New Harbinger Publications, 1989.

McMahon, S. *The Portable Therapist: Wise and Inspiring Answers to the Questions People in Therapy Ask Most*. New York: Dell Publishing, 1994.

Marmorstein J., and N. Marmorstein. *Awakening From Depression*. Santa Barbara, CA: Woodbridge Press, 1992.

Moyers, B. *Healing And The Mind*. New York: Doubleday, 1993.

Peck, S. *Further Along The Road Less Traveled: The Unending Journey Toward Spiritual Growth*. New York: Simon & Schuster, 1993.

————. *The Road Less Traveled: A New Psychology of Love, Traditional, Values and Spiritual Growth*. New York: Simon & Schuster, 1978.

Peterson, C. and L. M. Bossio. *Health and Optimism*. New York: The Free Press, 1991.

Porat, F. *Creative Life Management: Stress Reduction for an Enhanced Quality of Life*. Menlo Park, CA: NewLife Books, 1995.

Roger, J., and P. McWilliams. *You Can't Afford The Luxury Of A Negative Thought: A Book For People With Any Life-Threatening Illness–Including Life*. Los Angeles, CA: Prelude Press, 1991.

Sher, B., with A. Gottlieb. *How To Get What You Really Want: A Unique, Step-By-Step Plan To Pinpoint Your Goals & Make Your Dreams Come True*. N.Y.: Ballantine, 1979.

Tavris, C. *Anger: The Misunderstood Emotion*. New York: Simon & Schuster, 1989.

Whitfield, C. L. *Healing The Child Within: Discovery And Recovery For Adult Children Of Dysfunctional Families*. Deerfield Beach, FL: HealthCommunication, 1989.

Whittaker, T. C. *The Inner Path: From Where You Are To Where You Want To Be*. New York: Fawcett Crest Books, Ballantine Books, 1986.

Yoder, B. *The Recovery Resource Book: The Best Available Information on Addictions and Codependence*. New York: Simon & Schuster, 1990.

Spirituality Books

Cousineau, P. *Soul: An Archaeology: Readings from Socrates to Ray Charles.* San Francisco: Harper San Francisco, 1994.

Dossey, L. *Healing Words: The Power of Prayer and The Practice of Medicine.* San Francisco: Harper San Francisco, 1993.

———. *Recovering the Soul: A Scientific & Spiritual Search.* N.Y.: Bantam Books, 1989.

Foundation For Inner Peace. *A Course In Miracles.* Tiburon, CA: Foundation For Inner Peace, 1976.

Goldsmith, J. S. *The Art of Meditation.* S. F., CA: HarperSan Francisco, 1990.

Jafolla, R., and M.A. *The Quest: A Journey of Spiritual Rediscovery.* Unity Village, MO: 1993. (To order, write: Unity School, Unity Village, MO 64065.)

Moore, T. *Care of the Soul: A Guide for Cultivating Depth & Sacredness in Everyday Life.* New York: Harper Collins, 1992.

Taylor, T. L. *Messengers of Light.* Tiburon, CA: H.J. Kramer, 1990.

Williamson, M. *A Return To Love.* New York: Harper Perennial, 1993.

Zukav, G. *The Seat of the Soul.* New York: Simon & Schuster, 1994.

Weight Control Books

Arterburn, S., M. Ehemann, and V. Lamphear. *Gentle Eating: Permanent Weight Loss Through Gradual Life Changes. A Proven Weight-Loss Program for Those Who Want to Lose 25 Pounds or More.* Nashville, Thomas Nelson Publ., 1994.

Chopra, D. *Perfect Weight: The complete mind/body program for achieving and maintaining your ideal weight.* New York: Harmony Books, 1994.

Helmstetter, S., with B. Schwartz. *Self-Talk For Weight Loss: Lose Weight, Keep It Off, And Never Diet Again*. Breakthru Publishing, 1994.

McClernan, J. *Change Your Mind, Change Your Weight*. Phoenix, AZ: Health Plus Publishers, 1985.

McDougall, J. A., and M. McDougall. *The McDougall Program For Maximum Weight Loss*. New York: Dutton, Penguin Books, 1994.

Ornish, D. *Eat More, Weigh Less: Life Choice Program For Losing Weight Safely While Eating Abundantly*. (With heart-healthy recipes.) N.Y.: HarperCollins, 1993.

Overeaters Anonymous. *The Twelve Steps and Twelve Traditions of Overeaters Anonymous*. Torrance, CA: Overeaters Anonymous, Inc., 1993. (Write: O.A., 383 Van Ness Ave., Suite 1601, Torrance, CA 90501. Or call: (310) 618-8835.

Powter, S. *Food*. New York: Simon & Schuster, 1995.

————. *The Pocket Powter: Questions and Answers to Help You Change the Way You Look and Feel Forever*. New York: Simon & Schuster, 1994.

————. *Stop the Insanity: Eat, Breathe, Move*. New York: Simon & Schuster, 1993.

Ray, S. *The Only Diet There Is*. Berkeley, CA: Celestial Arts, 1981.

Sundermeyer, C. A. *Emotional Weight: Change Your Relationship With Food By Changing Your Relationship With Yourself*. New York: Perigee Books, 1993.

University of California at Berkeley. *The Wellness Lowfat Cookbook*. New York: Rebus, Inc. Distributed by Random House, 1989.

Note To Reader:

Feel free to submit any of your own health tips, suggestions, experiences, resources, references, or anything else that has helped you to cope with chronic illness. If any of your ideas or resources are included in future editions of this book, I will be happy to give you credit for them.

Please send your suggestions and/or comments to:

Pamela D. Jacobs • 750 La Playa, Suite 647 • San Francisco, CA 94121

<u>Order Form (OK to photocopy this form)</u>
<u>Books by Pamela D. Jacobs, M.A.</u>

	Quantity	**Unit Price**	**Total**
1. *500 Tips For Coping With Chronic Illness*	_____	$11.95	_____
2. *Chronic Fatigue Syndrome:*			
How To Find Facts & Get Help	_____	$9.95	_____

Subtotal: $_____

California residents please add 8.5% sales tax: $_____

$2.50 shipping for first book & $1.00 for each additional book: $_____

Total: $_____

To help save postage and paper, please send payment with all orders. Thank you. Please include your complete mailing address and telephone number with your order.

Order from: **Pamela Jacobs, 750 La Playa, Suite 647, San Francisco, CA 94121**

Order Form (OK to photocopy this form)
Books by Robert D. Reed Publishers

		Quantity	Unit Price	Total
1.	*500 Tips For Coping With Chronic Illness* by Pamela D. Jacobs, M.A.	_____	$11.95	_____
2.	*Chronic Fatigue Syndrome: How To Find Facts & Get Help* by Pamela D. Jacobs, M.A.	_____	$9.95	_____
3.	*50 Things You Can Do About Guns* by James M. Murray	_____	$7.95	_____
4.	*The Funeral Book* by Clarence W. Miller	_____	$7.95	_____
5.	*Get Out Of Your Thinking Box* by Lindsay Collier	_____	$7.95	_____

Subtotal: $_____

California residents please add 8.5% sales tax: $_____

$2.50 shipping for first book & $1.00 for each additional book: $_____

Total: $_____

To help save postage and paper, please send payment with all orders. Thank you.
Please include your complete mailing address and telephone number with your order.

Robert D. Reed Publishers, 750 La Playa, Suite 647, San Francisco, CA 94121

About The Author

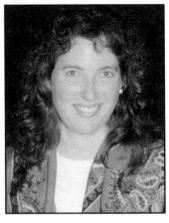

Pamela D. Jacobs, M.A. is a freelance writer/editor and creative director for Robert D. Reed Publishers in San Francisco. She is working toward a degree in holistic and environmental health, and she is planning to become a certified health educator. Pamela holds a B.A. in foods and nutrition and an M.A. in professional, technical, and museum writing from San Francisco State University, where she helped to write and edit several museum exhibit catalogs. She has also written and edited screenplays, scripts, health care materials, marketing brochures, training manuals, and advertising copy. Her book, *Chronic Fatigue Syndrome: How To Find Facts And Get Help* (1992), helps people to cope with a highly debilitating and devastating illness.

Coping with a chronic illness for many years herself has given Pamela first-hand awareness of just how challenging illness can be. Still, she maintains hope, optimism, and a healthy sense of humor. She has attended numerous health classes and medical conferences, consulted with physicians and psychotherapists for advice on coping, answered hundreds of hotline calls, and attended and facilitated support groups for people with health problems.

Healing Perspectives

Life is full of intricate miracles, both visible and invisible...

From the way your body functions to the beauty you find in nature.

Open to life's miracles, such as healing angels or the power of prayer.

Observe how your life's puzzle pieces fit together, giving meaning to madness.

See how your personal journey has brought you to this moment in time.

What are common themes of your life experiences, lessons, and dreams?

Use these to work through any emotional pain, anger, envy, or regret.

Forgive yourself and others. Release your past and live right now.

Create inner and outer strength, guidance, harmony, and balance.

Enjoy life's treasures, such as a bird's song or a child's laughter.

Develop a deeper sense of yourself. Love and appreciate who you are.

Trust your intuition. Think of yourself as "perfection in progress."

– Pamela D. Jacobs